"Living ... Without Milk"

Read What the Experts Say

"NOT EVERYONE CAN LOVE ELSIE THE COW. More than 20 percent of the population suffer from lactose intolerance ... 'Living ... Without Milk' is a cookbook and nutritional guide which offers over 100 nonmilk recipes besides lists of substitute foods that will replace the nutrients lost in abstaining from milk and milk products. Author Jacqueline Hostage tells readers how to determine if they suffer from that intolerance and cautions against food additives that contribute to the problem."

"The Detroit News"

"This is a timely book as more and more doctors are urging us to forego the three glasses of milk per day."

Allergy Information Association , Canada

"'Living ... Without Milk' is a good basic non-milk cookbook with some very interesting ideas presented."

Dr. Grace M. Anderson

"The Chairman of the Subcommittee on Information Services has approved your book, 'Living . . . Without Milk'."

Allergy Foundation of America

LIVING ... WITHOUT MILK

by Jacqueline E. Hostage

With Illustrations by Robin Hostage

Betterway Publications

New York

LIBRARY OF CONGRESS CATALOG CARD NUMBER: 78-72504

ISBN: 0-932620-02-7

Second printing April 1979

Printed in the United States of America

CONTENTS

2051792

ACKNOWLEDGEMENT

is gratefully made to the General Foods Corporation and the Rich Products Corporation for some
of the special recipes used in this book. These
sources are identified by the following abbrevi-
ations printed to the right of each recipe:

General Foods Corporation $\begin{pmatrix} GF \end{pmatrix}$
Rich Products Corporation $\begin{pmatrix} R \end{pmatrix}$

* Indicates that recipe appears elsewhere in
   the book. Please check Recipe Index, p.91

INTRODUCTION: DEFINING THE PROBLEM

Milk is a wholesome, nutritious product which most of us have grown to accept as an essential part of our daily diet. For some of us, however, milk can produce reactions which range from a slight sniffle or "just a little gas pain" to acute asthma or debilitating, chronic diarrhea.

The medical literature concerning symptoms attributed to milk allergy or sensitivity includes: abdominal swelling, spastic colon, nausea, vomiting, constipation, diarrhea, mucus colitis, canker sores, runny nose, chronic cough, nasal congestion, ear infections, eczema, irritability, swollen and painful joints, iron-deficiency anemia, and even hidden bleeding in babies from injuries to the intestinal tract.

Some individuals have a true allergy and have a specific allergic reaction to milk in any form; others are milk intolerant and their systems lack the enzyme (lactase) which is necessary to digest the milk sugar (lactose) in the milk. The symptoms may vary but the villain is the same - milk.

Dr. Frederic Speer of the Speer Allergy Clinic in Shawnee Mission, Kansas is quoted in an Associated Press release as stating that, "In the United States, cow's milk is the most common allergen". To add to the many who are allergic to milk, there are the millions who become sensitive to milk as their bodies stop producing the enzyme that enables them to digest the milk sugar in milk or milk products. A United Press International release of August, 1976 reports that Dr. Clinton Lillibridge, head of the gastroenterology unit at Genesee Hospital in Rochester, New York finds that "many humans lose their ability to digest milk sometime after the age of weaning". He explains that the "milk sugar or lactose stays in the intestines and ferments. It attracts water, causes the bowels to distend and results in gas, bloating, cramps, and diarrhea". To point up the magnitude of the problem, he estimates that "one in every five white Americans" is lactase deficient and that "about three-quarters of all Negro Americans and as many as 90 percent of Indians and Orientals lose their milk tolerance with age". Dr. Lillibridge adds that "internists and general practitioners are usually unaware of the high incidence of milk intolerance".

How do you find out if milk is your problem? In the case of an allergy, the most common method used is to keep a careful record of all foods eaten along with the notation of any symptoms of allergy. This, followed by the elimination of milk and milk products from the diet and the subsequent relief of the symptoms, may identify an allergy to milk. The determination of a milk sugar sensitivity can be made through the use of a simple and reliable lactose tolerance blood test which measures the blood sugar level at fasting and again at various intervals over a period of several hours.

Avoiding milk is not difficult once you become familiar with all of its varied forms.

While cheese and yogurt readily come to mind as milk products, cow's milk contains lactose, whey, lactalbumin, casein and dozens of other natural chemicals, some of which form the basis for additives that we find in other foods.

The purpose of this book is not only to help you prepare more interesting meals without using milk or milk products but to help you identify the "hidden" ingredients that contribute to the problem. Consider that additives used in this country amount to more than three pounds of food additives per person per year and that the use of additives is climbing each year. Your doctor can help you decide which foods and additives you should avoid after he has determined the nature and the extent of your problem. Knowing exactly what is in everything you eat will be a challenge that becomes easier as you familiarize yourself with the ingredients in your favorite products and as you prepare more dishes using only basic, milk-free ingredients.

Finally, don't be discouraged if you don't find immediate relief, particularly if you have a lactose sensitivity. It may take several weeks to cleanse your system of the undigested milk that has accumulated and for your digestion to return to normal.

MILK-FREE DIET - FOODS TO AVOID

BEVERAGES: Made with milk or chocolate or cocoa preparations containing milk.

BAKED GOODS: All breads prepared with milk or milk products. Most commercial breads - except Kosher - contain milk or milk products. Soda crackers (check labels), doughnuts, popovers, pancakes, waffles, rusk, many crackers and cookies.

BREADED FOODS: Any containing milk or crumbs from bread, crackers, or cereal containing milk or milk products.

CEREALS: Any prepared with milk or containing milk or milk products. Check dry cereal package labels carefully.

DESSERTS: Cakes, cookies, puddings, or pie crusts made with milk. Bavarian creams, blancmanges, custards, junket, ice cream, milk sherbet. Prepared mixes containing milk or milk products. Some commercial fruit fillings (check labels).

EGGS: Scrambled or creamed. Souffles.

FATS AND SALAD DRESSINGS: Butter, margarine made with milk or butter added. Salad dressings or boiled dressings containing milk, cream, butter, margarine, or cheese.

FRUITS: Canned or frozen prepared with lactose.

MEATS, POULTRY, FISH, SEAFOOD: Any prepared with milk or milk products. Many commercial dinners, hamburgers, frankfurters, sausages, and cold cuts - except Kosher - contain dry milk or other milk products.

MILK AND MILK PRODUCTS: Fresh, whole, and skim milk. Condensed, evaporated, dried milk, and milk solids. Cultured and buttermilk. Sweet or sour cream. Butter. All Cheeses. Powdered and malted milk. Powdered coffee creamer (check labels). Curds, wheys, casein*, sodium caseinate*, and lactalbumin*.

SAUCES AND GRAVIES: White, cream, butter or hard sauces or gravies made with milk or milk products or any prepared dish using these sauces.

SOUPS: Canned, homemade, or dried mixes containing milk or milk products.

VEGETABLES: Creamed or scalloped; potatoes that have been mashed with milk or cream.

MISCELLANEOUS: Creamed or scalloped foods; any dipped in milk or butter or fried in butter; any prepared with cheese. Any prepared mixes containing milk or milk products. Caramels, toffee, butterscotch, chocolate or any other candy containing milk or milk products.

The above is a compilation of foods listed by most authorities. Below is a list of foods that appear on some lactose-free diets and it is included for your information:

DISCUSS WITH YOUR DOCTOR: Cocoa, chocolate, some instant coffee; chewing gum, powdered soft drinks, molasses, mono-sodium glutamate, party dips, blended spices, some dietetic and diabetic preparations. Cordials and liqueurs. Some medicines and vitamins. Sweetbreads, liver, brains. Corn, beets, peas, lima beans.

* These additives are from the protein of cow's milk and are permissible for those who cannot tolerate lactose (milk sugar) but not for those who are allergic to milk.

PRODUCTS TO CHECK CAREFULLY

BREADS may contain milk, milk products, molasses or whey.

BREAD CRUMBS may contain the same ingredients as bread without being specifically identified on the label. In addition, they may contain mixed spices, cheese or mono-sodium-glutamate. The same cautions apply to CROUTONS.

CANDIES, especially filled candy bars, should be checked carefully.

COLD CUTS, FRANKFURTERS, AND SAUSAGES may contain milk or milk products.

COOKIES AND CRACKERS often contain milk, butter, whey, or lactose.

DELICATESSEN MEATS, such as roast beef or corned beef, may have been prepared using a tenderizer containing mono-sodium-glutamate.

FAST FOOD hamburgers, frankfurters, fried chicken, or fried fish may contain dried milk used as an extender or have milk in the batter.

FROZEN FOODS. Vegetables in sauces, hamburgers, t.v. dinners, baked goods - all may contain milk or milk products. Even fruit may be sweetened with lactose.

"KOSHER" FOODS are generally acceptable but watch for foods identified as "kosher" but with the additional word "dairy" which means that they contain dairy products (and under Jewish dietary laws can be eaten only with dairy meals). "Kosher" foods are usually identified by a "K" (alone or in a circle); with a "U" in a circle; or by a "P" or the word "Parve".

MAYONNAISE may contain mono-sodium-glutamate.

MIXED SPICES often contain lactose as a binder
    or mono-sodium-glutamate as a flavor enhancer.

MIXES OF ALL TYPES should be checked carefully -
    including: pudding and dessert mixes; bread,
    cake, and cookie mixes; rice mixes and
    seasoned coating mixes; and pancake, muffin,
    or biscuit mixes.

"NON-DAIRY" products such as powdered or liquid
    creamers and powdered or frozen whipped
    toppings should all be checked carefully -
    some contain sodium caseinate, lactose, or
    whey solids.

PRESERVES AND JAMS occasionally have butter or
    margarine added to prevent the product from
    foaming during the manufacturing process.

RESTAURANTS are often heavy on the use of mono-
    sodium-glutamate, as well as, butter and
    cream.

VITAMINS AND MEDICINES frequently use lactose
    as a binder. Often, this is not listed on
    the label so you should ckeck with your doctor
    or write directly to the pharmaceutical comp-
    any.

WHEN INQUIRING ABOUT A PRODUCT, ALWAYS ASK: DOES
THIS PRODUCT CONTAIN BUTTER, MARGARINE, CHEESE
OF ANY KIND, FRESH MILK, DRIED OR POWDERED MILK,
CONDENSED OR EVAPORATED MILK, BUTTERMILK, FRESH
OR SOUR CREAM, YOGHURT, OR ANY MILK-DERIVED FOOD
ADDITIVE?

THE BETTER
BREAKFAST

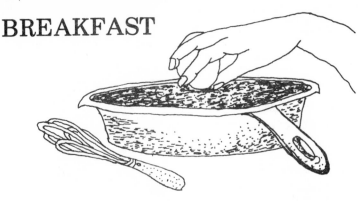

BREAKFAST COOKIES

1¼ cups unsifted FLOUR

2/3 cup SUGAR

½ cup POST® GRAPE-NUTS® Brand Cereal

1 teaspoon BAKING POWDER

½ pound BACON, cooked and crumbled

½ cup MILK-FREE MARGARINE

1 EGG

2 tablespoons frozen ORANGE JUICE concentrate, thawed, undiluted

1 tablespoon grated ORANGE PEEL

Combine dry ingredients; mix well. Add bacon, margarine, egg, orange juice concentrate, and orange peel. Mix until well blended. Drop by level tablespoons 2 inches apart on ungreased baking sheet.

Bake 10-12 minutes in a 350° oven or until edges of cookies are lightly browned but cookies are still soft.

Makes 2½ dozen.

PUFFED OMELET (CR)

For <u>each</u> serving:

2 EGGS

¼ cup COFFEE RICH®

SALT and PEPPER to taste

2 tablespoons MILK-FREE MARGARINE

FILLING: Sauteed mushrooms, bacon,
jelly, or catsup

Separate eggs. Add Coffee Rich® and seasonings
to yolks; beat until well mixed. Beat the egg
whites until stiff. Fold into the yolks. Melt
margarine in 8-inch skillet; add eggs. Cook,
loosening and lifting the edges until eggs are
set but still moist on top. Spread the eggs with
filling, reserving some for garnish. With a
rubber spatula roll the omelet away from you and
make the final roll by turning the omelet onto
serving dish. Garnish with reserved filling.

PANCAKES

1¼ cups sifted FLOUR

2½ teaspoons BAKING POWDER

2 tablespoons SUGAR

¾ teaspoon SALT

4 EGGS, separated

¾ cup WATER

3 tablespoons MILK-FREE MARGARINE (melted)

Sift together dry ingredients. Combine egg yolks
and water; add to dry ingredients mixing only
until dry ingredients are moist. Beat egg whites
until stiff; fold beaten egg whites and margarine
into batter. Cook on lightly greased griddle.

Makes 16 4-inch pancakes using ¼ cup batter each.

CRANBERRY NUT MUFFINS

1½ cups unsifted FLOUR

½ cup SUGAR

1 teaspoon BAKING POWDER

½ teaspoon SALT

½ teaspoon BAKING SODA

⅓ cup chopped NUTS

2 tablespoons ORANGE JUICE

1 tablespoon SALAD OIL

1 EGG, slightly beaten

1 8-oz. can WHOLE BERRY CRANBERRY SAUCE

Combine dry ingredients. Add remaining ingredients and stir until dry ingredients are evenly moistened. Fill muffin pans 2/3 full. Bake 15-20 minutes in a 400° oven. Makes 12.

QUICK APPLESAUCE MUFFINS

1 tablespoon SUGAR

½ teaspoon CINNAMON

1 cup unsifted FLOUR

6 tablespoons SUGAR

½ teaspoon SALT

½ teaspoon BAKING SODA

½ teaspoon CINNAMON

½ cup RAISINS

¼ cup chopped NUTS

½ cup APPLESAUCE

¼ cup OIL

½ teaspoon VANILLA

1 EGG

Combine the 1 tablespoon sugar and ½ teaspoon cinnamon; set aside. Combine remaining ingredients; blend at low speed 1 minute and beat at medium speed 1 minute. Fill muffin pans 2/3 full. Sprinkle reserved sugar and cinnamon over tops. Bake 15-20 minutes in a 400° oven or until done. Makes 12 muffins.

ORANGE CRUMB COFFEE CAKE

½ cup firmly packed BROWN SUGAR

½ cup finely chopped NUTS

½ teaspoon CINNAMON

½ teaspoon NUTMEG

2 cups sifted FLOUR

3 teaspoons BAKING POWDER

1 teaspoon SALT

¼ cup granulated SUGAR

⅓ cup SHORTENING

1 EGG, slightly beaten

¾ cup ORANGE JUICE

2 tablespoons MILK-FREE MARGARINE

Melt margarine and set aside to cool. Combine brown sugar, nuts, and spices; set aside. Combine flour, baking powder, salt, and granulated sugar in bowl; cut in shortening until mixture resembles coarse meal. Add egg and orange juice, stir until blended. Drop mixture by heaping tablespoonfuls into sugar-nut mixture, shaping into balls and coating well. Place balls in greased 8-inch square pan. Sprinkle with remaining sugar mixture and drizzle with the melted margarine.

Bake 30-35 minutes in a 375° oven. Serve warm.

. . . Combine any of these beverages with delicious "Breakfast Cookies"* for a nutritious
breakfast or snack . . .

CREAMY "SHAKE"

½ cup non-dairy CREAMER

½ cup ICE WATER

1 teaspoon SUGAR

¼ cup mashed STRAWBERRIES

1 tablespoon VANILLA INSTANT PUDDING

Shake in jar or blend in blender. Let stand a
minute before serving.
Makes 1 serving.

NOTE: In place of the strawberries, try substituting any one of the following: 2 tablespoons
strawberry or raspberry jam, 1 tablespoon
instant coffee, or 2 tablespoons chocolate
or carob syrup.

FRESH FRUIT SMOOTHIE

1 cup PINEAPPLE JUICE

1 cup ORANGE JUICE

1 PEACH, cut up (optional)

1 BANANA, cut up

2 cracked ICE CUBES

1 tablespoon SUGAR

Omit peach and mash banana if not using blender.
Shake in jar or blend in blender.
Makes 3 servings.

GOLDEN EGGNOG

$\frac{1}{4}$ cup non-dairy CREAMER

1 EGG

$\frac{1}{2}$ cup ORANGE JUICE

2 teaspoons SUGAR

Mix well with egg beater or blend in blender.
Makes 1 serving.

BANANA FLIP

$\frac{3}{4}$ cup non-dairy CREAMER

$\frac{3}{4}$ cup ICE WATER

2 teaspoons SUGAR

1 ripe BANANA (cut up or mashed)

2 tablespoons LEMON INSTANT PUDDING

Mash banana if not using blender. Shake in jar
or blend in blender. Let stand a minute before
serving.
Makes 2 servings.

"CHOCOLATE" SYRUP

1 cup SUGAR

$\frac{1}{2}$ cup COCOA or CAROB POWDER

1 cup WATER

$\frac{1}{2}$ teaspoon VANILLA

Combine sugar, cocoa or carob powder, and water
in saucepan. Bring to boil and simmer 5 minutes
or until ingredients are blended. Add vanilla.

PACKAGED PRODUCT INGREDIENTS ARE LIKE THE WEATHER
--- ALWAYS CHANGING. READ THE LABEL EVERY TIME
YOU BUY A PRODUCT.

APPETIZERS & DIPS

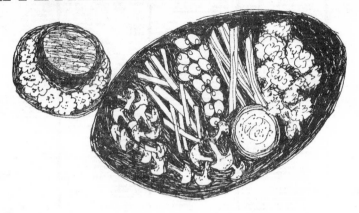

SEAFOOD REMOULADE

2 6-ounce packages FROZEN COOKED SHRIMP

½ cup CELERY, finely diced

¼ cup MAYONNAISE

2 tablespoons SWEET PICKLE RELISH

2 tablespoons CHILI SAUCE

2 teaspoons WORCESTERSHIRE SAUCE

Thaw and drain shrimp. Combine with remaining ingredients; blend well. Chill.

VARIATION: Substitute 2 6-ounce packages frozen cooked SHRIMP AND CRAB MEAT or 1 20-ounce can drained CHICK PEAS.

NOTE: These make delightful luncheon salads with the addition of more celery and mayonnaise. Serve on lettuce.

23

BAKED CLAMS OREGANO

4 tablespoons MILK-FREE MARGARINE

2 tablespoons minced ONION

1 clove GARLIC, minced

1 8-ounce can MINCED CLAMS and JUICE

1 teaspoon OREGANO

1 teaspoon PARSLEY FLAKES

½ cup SEASONED BREAD CRUMBS*

Saute onion and garlic in margarine until tender.
Add remaining ingredients, except bread crumbs;
simmer five minutes. Mix in bread crumbs; pile
lightly into baking shells. For added "zing",
sprinkle lightly with paprika. Fills about 12
2-inch shells.

Bake 15-20 minutes in a 375° oven or until tops
are lightly browned.

DIETER'S DELIGHT NIBBLERS

The day before serving, wash CAULIFLOWER and break
into bite-sized flowerets. Clean and cut CARROTS,
CELERY, and GREEN PEPPER into 2-inch sticks. Place
vegetables in a large container, alternating with
ICE CUBES and sprinkling with 1 tablespoon SALT.
Fill container with cold water, cover tightly, and
refrigerate. Just before serving, drain thoroughly
and arrange on tray with cleaned, chilled tiny
TOMATOES, RADISHES, and SCALLIONS. Serve with
TANGY VEGETABLE DIP.

TANGY VEGETABLE DIP

1 cup MAYONNAISE

¼ cup CATSUP

1 tablespoon CHILI SAUCE

2 teaspoons HORSERADISH

1 tablespoon LEMON JUICE

1 clove GARLIC, minced

Dash TABASCO

Combine all ingredients until smooth. Chill for several hours to blend flavors.

NOTE: Reduce or increase the mayonnaise to suit taste.

COCKTAIL MEATBALLS

1 pound GROUND BEEF

¼ cup milk-free dry BREAD CRUMBS*

1 medium ONION, Minced or grated

1 teaspoon SALT

1 EGG, beaten

1 cup CHILI SAUCE

2/3 cup GRAPE JELLY

1 tablespoon LEMON JUICE

Combine ground beef, bread crumbs, onion, salt, and egg; shape into 24-30 small balls. Combine remaining ingredients in shallow saucepan or skillet; heat, stirring until smooth. Drop in meatballs; simmer 20 minutes, covered. If sauce does not completely cover meatballs, turn or baste once during cooking to assure that they brown evenly.

SPICY MARINATED MUSHROOMS

1 pound fresh small MUSHROOMS

½ cup WINE VINEGAR

½ cup SALAD OIL

1 medium ONION, thinly sliced

1 clove GARLIC, minced

1 teaspoon SALT

1 tablespoon DRIED PARSLEY

1 teaspoon prepared MUSTARD

1 tablespoon BROWN SUGAR

Rinse mushrooms quickly or wipe with damp paper
towel; trim stems. Combine remaining ingredients
and bring to boil. Add mushrooms and simmer
gently 15 minutes. Chill several hours or overnight in covered bowl. Keeps several days. Drain
just before serving.

MARINATED ARTICHOKES

2 cups ARTICHOKE HEARTS, canned or frozen

2 tablespoons LEMON JUICE

2 tablespoons SALAD OIL

1 tablespoon SUGAR

1 tablespoon WATER

1 clove GARLIC, finely minced

¼ teaspoon dried OREGANO

If artichoke hearts are frozen, cook according to
package directions. Drain. Combine all ingredients in bowl. Cover tightly and chill several
hours or overnight. Drain; serve with picks.

NOTE: Leftover marinated mushrooms or artichokes
are delicious used in tossed green salad
with a plain Oil and Vinegar Dressing.

MAIN DISHES

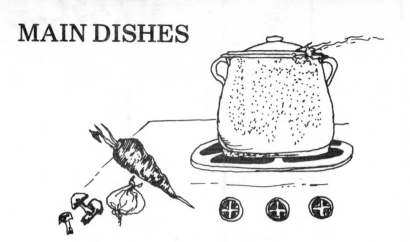

OVEN BEEF RAGOUT

2 pounds BEEF, cut for stew

3-4 CARROTS, cut in 1-inch pieces

1 cup chopped CELERY

2 ONIONS, sliced

3-4 POTATOES, pared and cut up

1 16-ounce can TOMATOES

1 8-ounce can TOMATO SAUCE

1 clove GARLIC

$\frac{1}{4}$ cup MINUTE® TAPIOCA

1 tablespoon SUGAR

$\frac{1}{2}$ cup DRY RED WINE (optional)

1 cup sliced WATER CHESTNUTS

$\frac{1}{4}$-$\frac{1}{2}$ pound sliced fresh MUSHROOMS

Combine all ingredients except water chestnuts and mushrooms in Dutch oven or large casserole. Cover.

Bake 5 hours in a 250° oven. Add water chestnuts and mushrooms during last hour of baking. Season to taste.

BARBECUED MEAT LOAVES

1 pound GROUND BEEF

1 EGG, slightly beaten

2 tablespoons milk-free BREAD CRUMBS

1 tablespoon ONION, minced

2 tablespoons WATER

1 teaspoon SALT

Dash PEPPER

$\frac{1}{3}$ cup CATSUP

2 tablespoons VINEGAR

$\frac{1}{4}$ teaspoon WORCESTERSHIRE SAUCE

$\frac{1}{2}$ teaspoon CHILI POWDER

1 tablespoon ONION, minced

Combine first seven ingredients; form into two
loaves. Place in shallow pan. Combine remaining
ingredients; spread on loaves.

Bake 35 minutes in 375° oven. Baste once or twice.

QUICK SAVORY MEAT LOAF (GF)

2 pounds GROUND BEEF

$\frac{1}{3}$ cup MINUTE® TAPIOCA

$\frac{1}{3}$ cup finely chopped ONION

$1\frac{1}{2}$ teaspoons SALT

$\frac{1}{4}$ teaspoon PEPPER

$\frac{1}{4}$ teaspoon SAVORY (optional)

1 12-ounce can TOMATOES, mashed

Combine all ingredients, mixing well. Spoon into
9x5-inch loaf pan. Press lightly.

Bake 1 to $1\frac{1}{4}$ hours in a 350° oven.

28

BEEF 'N PEPPER STEAK

1 pound BEEF TENDERLOIN, sliced $\frac{1}{4}$" thick

2 tablespoons SALAD OIL

1 medium ONION, sliced

1 large GREEN PEPPER, cut in 1" cubes

1 clove GARLIC, minced

1 cup BOUILLION OR BEEF BROTH

1 tablespoon SOY SAUCE

$1\frac{1}{2}$ tablespoons CORNSTARCH

$\frac{1}{4}$ cup WATER

2 small TOMATOES, cut into sections

Brown beef in oil. Push to one side. Add onion, pepper, garlic; cook five minutes or until vegetables are softened. Add bouillion, soy sauce, and cornstarch dissolved in the water. Cover; simmer ten minutes or until meat and vegetables are tender. Add tomatoes. Heat through. Serve with rice.

Makes 4 servings.

NOTE: Whole beef tenderloin can be a "bargain" when it's on special because there is so little waste. This is a good recipe to use up the thin end and the trimmings.

LABELS MAKE INTERESTING READING!!!

EASY POT ROAST

4 pound boneless POT ROAST

2 small ONIONS, chopped

1 small CARROT, diced

1 stalk CELERY, diced

2 teaspoons SALT

$\frac{1}{4}$ teaspoon PEPPER

1 BAYLEAF

$\frac{1}{2}$ cup TOMATO or SPAGHETTI SAUCE

Brown meat in pan over medium heat; place on large sheet of heavy duty foil. Brown vegetables in same pan; sprinkle on meat along with seasonings. Pour sauce over. Close foil, sealing edges with double folds to form airtight package. Place in shallow pan to catch any leaks.

Bake $3\frac{1}{2}$ hours in a 300° oven or 4 hours in a 250° oven.

SUPER-EASY POT ROAST

3 to 4 pound boneless POT ROAST

1 envelope ONION SOUP MIX

Place meat in center of long sheet of heavy duty foil. Sprinkle all sides of meat with onion soup mix. Close foil, sealing edges with double folds to form airtight package. Place in shallow pan.

Bake 3 hours in a 350° oven.

TOFU MANICOTTI

8 uncooked MANICOTTI SHELLS

1 small ONION, minced

1 clove GARLIC, minced

1 tablespoon MILK-FREE MARGARINE

2 cups crumbled TOFU (about two cakes)

2 teaspoons DRIED PARSLEY

1 EGG, slightly beaten

1 quart TOMATO SAUCE with MEAT
  (preferably homemade)

Cook manicotti shells according to package directions until tender; drain; allow to cool. Crumble and measure tofu; place on paper towel and let excess moisture drain while preparing remaining ingredients. Meanwhile, saute onion and garlic in margarine until onion is transparent. Combine sauteed onions and garlic, tofu, parsley, egg, and salt and pepper to taste. Fill shells with mixture. Pour half of the tomato sauce in the bottom of a shallow baking dish. Place stuffed shells in dish in a single layer; pour remaining sauce over the manicotti. Cover with aluminum foil. (May be refrigerated at this point for baking later if desired.)

Bake, covered, 40-45 minutes in a 350° oven.

NOTE: For family members not on a lactose-free diet, sliced mozarella cheese may be used on their portions. After baking, top part of the manicotti with the cheese, continue baking, uncovered, until cheese melts and is bubbly, about 5 minutes.

VERSATILE BAKED CHICKEN

4 small CHICKEN BREASTS, split and boned

½ cup MILK-FREE MARGARINE

2 tablespoons FLOUR

1 cup CORNFLAKE CRUMBS

1 teaspoon SALT

1 teaspoon ROSEMARY or OREGANO, crumbled

Melt margarine and blend in flour until smooth.
Dip chicken pieces in margarine mixture and coat
well with combined crumbs and seasonings. Place
on shallow baking pan and refrigerate if not
baking immediately.

Bake 45-60 minutes in a 350° oven.

NOTE: Crumbs will adhere better and be crisper
        if skin is removed from chicken. Any type
        of chicken parts can be used; if using
        boneless cutlets, use the shorter baking
        time but use the longer baking time when
        using large cutlets or bone-in chicken
        parts.

        Mayonnaise or barbecue sauce may be substi-
        tuted for the margarine and flour or a
        large clove of garlic, crushed, can be
        added to the margarine mixture. Seasoned
        dry bread crumbs or crushed potato chips
        can replace the cornflake crumbs.

        A very adaptable recipe that is equally
        delicious hot or cold and is particularly
        festive served with a sauce made by heating
        1¼ cups CREAM-OF-MUSHROOM SOUP SUBSTITUTE*
        with ½ cup dry white wine.

CHICKEN-MACARONI CASSEROLE

3 pounds CHICKEN PARTS, cut-up

$\frac{1}{4}$ cup FLOUR

$\frac{1}{2}$ teaspoon SALT

$\frac{1}{4}$ teaspoon PEPPER

$\frac{1}{4}$ cup COOKING OIL

$\frac{1}{2}$ cup chopped ONION

$\frac{1}{4}$ cup chopped GREEN PEPPER

1 clove GARLIC, minced

3 CARROTS, sliced

3 stalks CELERY, sliced

1 16-ounce can TOMATO SAUCE

1 cup WATER

$1\frac{1}{2}$ cups ELBOW MACARONI, uncooked

Shake chicken in plastic bag containing flour, salt, and pepper. Brown in heated oil in skillet. Remove from pan and lightly saute onion, pepper, and garlic. Add remaining ingredients, except macaroni, and simmer 10 minutes. Put macaroni in large, lightly greased casserole; cover with chicken pieces, pour sauce over all. Cover.

Bake $1\frac{1}{2}$ hours in a 325° oven.

SKILLET HERB CHICKEN

3 pounds CHICKEN PARTS, cut-up

$\frac{1}{4}$ cup FLOUR

$\frac{3}{4}$ teaspoon SALT

$\frac{1}{4}$ teaspoon PEPPER

$\frac{1}{4}$ cup SHORTENING

$1\frac{1}{4}$ cups CREAM-OF-MUSHROOM SOUP SUBSTITUTE*

$\frac{1}{2}$ cup WATER (part white wine, if desired)

1 medium ONION, sliced

$\frac{1}{2}$ teaspoon THYME

Coat chicken with flour and seasonings; brown in heated shortening in skillet. Add soup, water; top with onion slices, thyme. Simmer, covered, basting often for 30 minutes or until tender.

Makes 4 servings.

PORK CHOP SKILLET DINNER

4 PORK CHOPS

3 medium ONIONS, sliced

3 raw POTATOES, sliced

DRY MUSTARD

$1\frac{1}{2}$ cups drained CANNED TOMATOES

Brown chops in pan and remove. Rub thoroughly with dry mustard. Brown the onions in the same pan; cover with the sliced potatoes, the pork chops. Cover with the tomatoes; season to taste with salt and pepper. Simmer for one hour or until chops and potatoes are tender.

Makes 4 servings.

34

CREAMY SCALLOP CASSEROLE

1 pound BAY SCALLOPS
   (or cut up Sea Scallops)

1 EGG YOLK, beaten

$\frac{1}{4}$ cup liquid NON-DAIRY CREAMER

1 teaspoon LEMON JUICE

2 tablespoons VERMOUTH (or white wine)

1 tablespoon ONION, minced

$\frac{1}{2}$ teaspoon SALT

Dash PEPPER   **2051792**

3/4 cup fresh MILK-FREE BREAD CRUMBS

1 tablespoon MILK-FREE MARGARINE, melted

Place scallops in bottom of shallow 1-quart baking dish. Combine egg yolk, creamer, lemon juice,
vermouth and seasonings; pour over scallops.
Combine bread crumbs and margarine and sprinkle
over top of casserole.

Bake 30 minutes in a 350° oven; raise heat to
450° for a few minutes more to brown crumbs.

CRUNCHY TUNA BAKE

1 6$\frac{1}{2}$-ounce can TUNA, drained

4 ounces WIDE EGG NOODLES

1$\frac{1}{4}$ cups CREAM-OF-MUSHROOM SOUP SUBSTITUTE*

1 4-ounce package POTATO CHIPS

2 hard cooked EGGS (optional), quartered

Cook noodles as directed on package and drain well.
Reserve enough potato chips for top of casserole;
crush remaining chips and cover bottom of shallow
1$\frac{1}{2}$ quart casserole. Combine remaining ingredients;
turn into casserole; top with chips.

Bake 20 minutes in 350° oven or until bubbly.

OVEN FRIED FISH FILLETS

1½ pounds COD or HADDOCK, fresh or frozen

2 tablespoons LEMON JUICE

¼ cup FLOUR

½ teaspoon SALT

½ cup milk-free MARGARINE, melted

1 cup CORNFLAKE CRUMBS

Thaw fillets if frozen. Rinse, pat dry, and cut
into serving portions. Combine lemon juice, flour,
salt, and margarine, stirring into a smooth paste.
Dip fish in paste; coat well with cornflake crumbs.
Arrange in single layer on foil-lined baking pan.

Bake 20 minutes in a 400° oven or until fish flakes
easily with a fork.

Makes 6 servings.

SEVEN SEAS CASSEROLE

1¼ cups CREAM-OF-MUSHROOM SOUP SUBSTITUTE*

1¼ cups WATER (part creamer, if desired)

¼ teaspoon SALT

¼ cup chopped ONION (optional)

1⅓ cups MINUTE® RICE

1 6½ ounce can TUNA, SALMON, or LOBSTER

1 box thawed FROZEN PEAS

Combine soup, water, onion, and salt; bring to
boil. Pour half into greased 1½ quart casserole.
In layers, add Minute® Rice, seafood, peas. Pour
over remaining soup; sprinkle with paprika, if
desired. Cover.

Bake 20 minutes in a 375° oven.

TUNA-TOFU LOAF

1 6½-ounce can TUNA, drained

3 EGGS, slightly beaten

¼ cup milk-free dry BREAD CRUMBS

1 small ONION, minced

1 tablespoon DRIED PARSLEY

½ cup TOMATO SAUCE

½ teaspoon SALT

½ teaspoon BAKING POWDER

1 cup TOFU, crumbled (about ¼ pound)

Press tofu to remove excess moisture. Crumble or shred and measure; place on paper towel to drain any additional moisture while preparing remaining ingredients. In mixing bowl, flake tuna and combine with remaining ingredients except tofu. Fold in tofu gently but thoroughly. Pour into greased 8x4-inch loaf pan, cover, and refrigerate for at least 1 hour (but no longer than 1 day).

Bake, uncovered, for 50 to 60 minutes in a 350° oven or until brown.

NOTE: For plain TUNA LOAF, substitute an additional can of tuna for the tofu.

CELERY-DILL SAUCE* or CREAM-OF-MUSHROOM SOUP SUBSTITUTE* (thinned with a little white wine) complement this very well.

HERBED MUSHROOM OMELET

½ pound MUSHROOMS, rinsed and dried

2 tablespoons ONION, minced

4 tablespoons milk-free MARGARINE

¼ teaspoon THYME or TARRAGON, crumbled

8 EGGS

½ teaspoon SALT

Dash black PEPPER

Slice mushrooms. Heat margarine in large skillet.
Add mushrooms and herb; saute five minutes, stirring occasionally. Beat eggs with salt and pepper
and pour over mushrooms in skillet. Cook over
medium heat. Loosen set portion with spatula and
tilt pan to let uncooked portion run underneath.
Cook until set but not dry.

SPANISH OMELET

½ cup chopped ONION

½ cup chopped GREEN PEPPER

½ cup thinly sliced CELERY

1 large TOMATO, diced and drained

¼ teaspoon SUGAR

SALT and PEPPER

6 EGGS, beaten

3 tablespoons MILK-FREE MARGARINE

Saute onion and pepper in 2 tablespoons of the
margarine, about 8 minutes or until almost tender
but not brown. Add celery and tomato; sprinkle
with seasonings. Cover and cook slowly about 5
minutes or until celery is tender. Uncover, raise
heat and cook to evaporate juices. Add remaining
margarine; pour in eggs and cook, stirring until
eggs have set.

ACCOMPANIMENTS

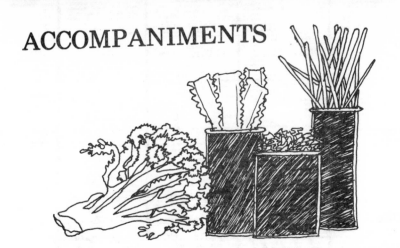

BAKED BEAN CASSEROLE

6 slices BACON, diced

1 large GREEN PEPPER, diced

2 medium ONIONS, chopped

½ pound MUSHROOMS, chopped

3 1-pound cans PORK AND BEANS
                   IN TOMATO SAUCE

¾ cup CHILI SAUCE

⅓ cup prepared MUSTARD

1 cup MAPLE SYRUP

1½ teaspoons OREGANO

5 WHOLE CLOVES

3 BAY LEAVES

Cook bacon until crisp and remove from pan. In remaining fat, saute green pepper, onions, and mushrooms until just tender. Add remaining ingredients; heat on top of stove just long enough to blend flavors. Serve immediately or store in refrigerator and reheat later by baking for 30 minutes in a 400° oven.

SAVORY TOMATOES

4 large, firm TOMATOES

2 cups fresh, milk-free BREAD CRUMBS

2 tablespoons DRIED PARSLEY

2 tablespoons chopped ONION

$\frac{1}{2}$ teaspoon SAGE or OREGANO

Dash PEPPER

$\frac{1}{4}$ cup MILK-FREE MARGARINE, melted

Core tomatoes and halve crosswise. Place cut side up on shallow, greased pan. Combine remaining ingredients; spread on tops of tomatoes.

Bake 10 minutes in a 450° oven.

Makes 8 servings.

BAKED CARROTS

1 pound CARROTS, pared

$\frac{1}{2}$ teaspoon SALT

1 teaspoon SUGAR

2 tablespoons milk-free MARGARINE

Cut carrots in halves or thirds, depending on size. Place in 1-quart casserole; sprinkle with salt and sugar; dot with margarine.

Bake $1\frac{1}{4}$ hours in a 325° oven or 1 hour in a 350° oven.

Makes 4 servings.

BONE MEAL IS A GOOD SOURCE OF CALCIUM

ZUCCHINI PROVENCAL

2 tablespoons milk-free MARGARINE

½ cup ONION, chopped

1 clove GARLIC, minced

4 medium ZUCCHINI, unpared

2 TOMATOES, peeled and chopped

1 teaspoon SALT

Dash pepper

¼ teaspoon OREGANO

Melt margarine in large skillet. Add onion and
garlic; cook five minutes or until tender. Slice
zucchini and add to skillet with remaining ingredients. Mix well, sprinkle with seasonings. Cover.
Cook over low heat about 15 minutes or just until
zucchini is tender but still crisp.

Makes 4 to 6 servings.

GREEN BEANS LUCETTE

1 9-ounce package frozen GREEN BEANS

1 3½-ounce can FRENCH-FRIED ONIONS

1¼ cups CREAM-OF-MUSHROOM SOUP SUBSTITUTE*

½ cup LIQUID from beans

Cook green beans according to directions on the
package; drain, reserving the ½ cup liquid.
Alternate layers of drained beans and onions in
shallow 1½ quart baking dish. Mix soup and liquid
and pour over vegetables.

Bake 30 minutes in a 350° oven or until bubbly.

Makes 4-6 servings.

SAN ANTONIO SPINACH PUDDING (R)

3 EGGS

1 cup COFFEE RICH®

1 tablespoon grated ONION

½ teaspoon SALT

¼ teaspoon PEPPER

1 10-ounce pkg. frozen CHOPPED SPINACH

Beat eggs until light and lemon colored. Blend in
Coffee Rich and seasonings. Cook spinach until
just tender, drain, and blend into Coffee Rich-
egg mixture. Pour into greased 1-quart casserole.

Bake 45 minutes in a 350° oven or until set and
silver knife comes out clean.

Makes 4 servings.

SAVORY OVEN-BAKED RICE

1 small ONION, finely chopped

⅓ cup chopped CELERY

¼ pound MUSHROOMS, chopped

3 tablespoons OIL

1½ cups uncooked REGULAR RICE

3 envelopes INSTANT CHICKEN BROTH

¼ teaspoon SAGE

¼ teaspoon BASIL

3½ cups BOILING WATER

Saute vegetables in oil until almost tender. Combine in 2-quart casserole with rice and seasonings. Pour boiling water over rice; stir with a
fork; cover.

Bake 45 minutes in a 350 oven. Fluff up rice
with a fork before serving.

42

SAVORY LEMON RICE (GF)

½ clove GARLIC, minced

2 tablespoons MILK-FREE MARGARINE

1⅓ cups MINUTE® RICE

1⅓ cups CHICKEN BROTH

½ teaspoon SALT

2 tablespoons chopped PARSLEY

1 tablespoon LEMON JUICE

1 teaspoon grated LEMON RIND

Saute garlic in margarine until golden brown. Stir
in rice, broth, and salt. Bring quickly to boil
over high heat. Cover, remove from heat, and let
stand 5 minutes. Add parsley, lemon juice, and
rind and fluff with a fork before serving. Serve
with fish, seafood, or chicken.

Makes 4 servings.

BARBECUE RICE (GF)

1⅓ cups WATER

½ teaspoon SALT

¼ teaspoon TABASCO SAUCE

1 teaspoon prepared MUSTARD

2 tablespoons minced ONION

2 tablespoons CHILI SAUCE

2 tablespoons MILK-FREE MARGARINE

1⅓ cups MINUTE® RICE

Combine all ingredients except rice in saucepan.
Bring to a boil. Stir in rice. Cover, remove
from heat, and let stand 5 minutes. Fluff with
fork before serving.

Makes 4 servings.

NOODLE RING

$\frac{1}{4}$ cup MILK-FREE MARGARINE, melted

1 pound WIDE NOODLES

4 EGGS, separated

1 teaspoon CINNAMON

$\frac{1}{4}$ teaspoon NUTMEG

$1\frac{1}{4}$ cups SUGAR

$\frac{1}{4}$ teaspoon SALT

1 cup RAISINS

$\frac{1}{2}$ cup chopped NUTS

Cook and drain noodles. Add margarine. Beat egg yolks with sugar; blend in seasonings. Fold lightly into noodles. Beat whites until stiff but not dry; fold into noodle mixture. Pour $\frac{1}{3}$ of mixture into greased 2-quart baking dish; sprinkle with half of the raisins and nuts; repeat; add remaining $\frac{1}{3}$ of mixture.

Bake 45 minutes in a 325° oven. Unmold or serve from dish.

NOTE: For an easy, no-pot-watching way to cook noodles (or spaghetti), just bring the required amount of water and salt to a full boil. Slowly drop in the noodles so that boiling doesn't stop. Stir and cover tightly. Remove from heat. Let stand 20 minutes.

"SINCE INGREDIENTS OF A PRODUCT MAY CHANGE, IT IS WISE TO CHECK THE INGREDIENTS LISTED ON THE PACKAGE EACH TIME A PRODUCT IS PURCHASED."
                                    General Foods Nutrition Services

SOUPS & SALADS

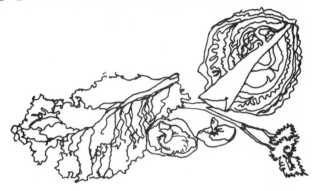

SPEEDY HAMBURGER-VEGETABLE SOUP

$\frac{1}{2}$ pound GROUND BEEF

1 large ONION, chopped

1 clove GARLIC, minced

4 cups BOILING WATER

4 BEEF BOUILLION CUBES

1 16-ounce can TOMATOES

$\frac{1}{2}$ cup diced CELERY

$\frac{1}{2}$ cup diced CARROTS

$\frac{1}{2}$ cup cut GREEN BEANS

1 tablespoon DRIED PARSLEY

1 BAYLEAF

SALT and PEPPER to taste

Brown ground beef, onion, and garlic lightly, adding oil if necessary. Add remaining ingredients; bring to boil and simmer 30-45 minutes or just until vegetables are done.

Makes 8 servings.

CREAM OF TOMATO SOUP

1 1-pound can TOMATOES

1 tablespoon ONION, minced

1 small BAYLEAF

1 teaspoon SUGAR

½ teaspoon SALT

Dash PEPPER

¾ cup WHITE SAUCE*

In saucepan, combine all ingredients <u>except</u> the White Sauce; simmer 10 minutes. (If desired, put through sieve or process in blender.) When ready to serve, stir in White Sauce gradually; heat through. Adjust seasonings and amount of White Sauce to taste.

NOTE: CREAM OF TOMATO SOUP combines very well with leftover CREAM-OF-MUSHROOM SOUP SUB-STITUTE* for a delicious TOMATO-MUSHROOM BISQUE. Thin with additional liquid non-dairy creamer if desired.

CREAM OF CELERY SOUP

1 cup CELERY, diced

¼ cup ONION, finely chopped

1 cup CHICKEN BROTH <u>or</u> WATER

1 cup WHITE SAUCE*

Cook celery and onion, covered, in chicken broth or salted water until tender (about 15 minutes). Stir in White Sauce. Heat through and season to taste.

Makes 3 servings.

NOTE: To make CELERY-DILL SAUCE, add an additional ½ cup WHITE SAUCE and 1 teaspoon (or to taste) DILL WEED. Heat through.

CLAM CHOWDER

2 tablespoons MILK-FREE MARGARINE

1 small ONION, chopped

1 small clove GARLIC, minced

½ small GREEN PEPPER, chopped

1 large CARROT, diced

1 TOMATO, peeled and chopped

1 large stalk CELERY, diced

1 large POTATO, diced

1 CHICKEN BOUILLION CUBE

Dash THYME

1 small BAYLEAF

1 8-oz. can MINCED CLAMS (broth included)

Saute onion, garlic, green pepper, and carrot in margarine until onion is golden and slightly tender. Add remaining ingredients except clams; simmer until vegetables are tender. Add clams and broth. Re-heat.

TUNA-MACARONI SALAD

1 cup uncooked ELBOW MACARONI

1 7-ounce can TUNA, drained

1 tablespoon grated ONION

1 tablespoon minced PARSLEY

¾ cup MAYONNAISE

½ teaspoon SALT

¼ teaspoon PEPPER

2 tablespoons SWEET PICKLE RELISH

Cook macaroni according to package directions; drain well and cool. Combine with remaining ingredients. Serve on lettuce.

47

HAM-RICE SALAD

1⅓ cups MINUTE® RICE

3 cups diced, cooked HAM

1 20-ounce can PINEAPPLE CHUNKS, drained

2 cups diced CELERY

½ cup diced GREEN PEPPER

1½ cups MAYONNAISE

1 teaspoon SALT

¼ teaspoon PEPPER

2 tablespoons LEMON JUICE

1 tablespoon grated ONION

1 tablespoon prepared MUSTARD

Cook rice according to package directions; cool. Add ham, pineapple, celery, and green pepper; chill. Combine remaining ingredients in separate bowl; chill. Just before serving, toss mixtures together lightly. Serve on lettuce.

CRANBERRY MOLD

1 3-oz. package JELL-O®, any red flavor

1 cup boiling WATER

¾ cup 7-UP or PINEAPPLE JUICE (canned)

1 8-oz. can WHOLE BERRY CRANBERRY SAUCE

1 cup diced APPLES or CELERY

½ cup coarsely chopped NUTS

Dissolve gelatin in boiling water. Add 7-Up or pineapple juice and cranberry sauce. Chill until slightly thickened. Stir in remaining ingredients and pour into 4-cup mold. Chill until firm.

NOTE: Recipe may be doubled; use only 1 cup 7-Up or pineapple juice.

CHERRY SALAD

1 17-ounce can SWEET DARK CHERRIES

1 3-ounce package JELL-O®, any red flavor

1 cup boiling WATER

2 tablespoons ORANGE JUICE

$\frac{3}{4}$ cup diced ORANGE SECTIONS

Drain cherries, reserving syrup; add cold water to syrup to make 1 cup liquid. Dissolve gelatin in the boiling water; add measured liquid and orange juice. Chill until the consistency of unbeaten egg whites. Fold in cherries and oranges. Pour into a 1-quart mold or individual molds. Chill until firm.

Makes 8 servings.

PINEAPPLE-LIME SALAD

1 3-oz. package LIME GELATIN

$\frac{3}{4}$ cup TOFU "SOUR CREAM"*

   or: 1 cup thawed COOL WHIP®

1 8-oz. can CRUSHED PINEAPPLE

$\frac{1}{2}$ cup CHOPPED PECANS

Drain pineapple, reserving liquid. Make gelatin using liquid plus enough water to make $1\frac{3}{4}$ cups. Chill until gelatin starts to thicken; fold in remaining ingredients. Pour into 4-cup mold. Chill until firm.

HAVE YOU READ ANY GOOD LABELS LATELY?

PINEAPPLE AND CARROT SALAD

1 3-oz. package LEMON GELATIN

1 cup boiling WATER

1½ cups PINEAPPLE JUICE

1 28-oz. can CRUSHED PINEAPPLE, drained

1 cup grated CARROTS

1 tablespoon VINEGAR

Dissolve gelatin in boiling water. Add pine-apple juice. Cool. Add remaining ingredients; stir. Pour into 1½ quart mold. Chill.

SWEET 'N SOUR COLESLAW

1 medium head CABBAGE, shredded

1 medium ONION, chopped

1 medium GREEN PEPPER, chopped

1 tablespoon SALT

1 cup VINEGAR

1½ cups SUGAR

1 teaspoon CELERY SEED

½ teaspoon MUSTARD SEED

Combine vegetables and salt in large pan. Cover with boiling water, cover pan and let stand for one hour. Drain well and return to pan. Heat vinegar, sugar and spices until sugar dissolves. Pour over vegetables; mix well. Store in glass container in refrigerator. Let flavors blend for a day before serving. Keeps for several weeks in refrigerator.

BAKED GOODS

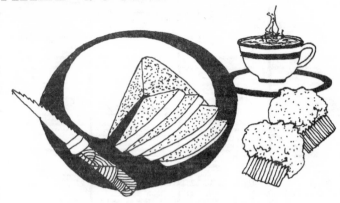

FEATHER-LITE BREAD

$\frac{1}{2}$ cup WARM WATER

2 packages DRY YEAST

6 EGGS, room temperature

$\frac{1}{4}$ cup SUGAR or HONEY

$\frac{1}{2}$ teaspoon SALT

5 cups white FLOUR

$\frac{1}{2}$ cup MILK-FREE MARGARINE, soft

Dissolve yeast in water and let stand until it
starts to bubble. Beat eggs until light and
lemon-colored; add sugar, salt, yeast and 3 cups
of the flour. Mix until smooth and elastic.
Add margarine and mix again until smooth. Blend
in remaining 2 cups flour with wooden spoon to
form a soft dough. Cover and let rise until
doubled.

Knead dough for 2 minutes on a well-floured sur-
face. Divide dough and shape into two loaves.
Place in two well-greased 9x5x3-inch loaf pans.
Let rise to top of pans.

Bake 35-40 minutes in a 400° oven.

COFFEE CAN RYE BREAD

1 package ACTIVE DRY YEAST

$\frac{1}{4}$ cup lukewarm WATER

$\frac{1}{2}$ cup BROWN SUGAR

1 teaspoon SALT

1 teaspoon CARAWAY SEED

1 tablespoon SHORTENING

2 cups WATER

3 cups unsifted FLOUR

2 cups LIGHT RYE FLOUR

Sprinkle active dry yeast over lukewarm water in cup and let stand until dissolved. Measure brown sugar into saucepan and add salt, caraway seed, shortening, and water. Bring to boil, lower heat and simmer gently for five minutes. Let cool to lukewarm and stir in dissolved yeast. Add unsifted flour and beat well. Transfer to greased bowl, cover with damp cloth and place in warm spot until dough has doubled in bulk. Stir down with spoon and blend in rye flour, mixing well. Spoon batter into three greased one pound coffee cans, filling about two-thirds. Place plastic cover over cans and let rise in warm spot until doubled in bulk.

Remove plastic covers. Bake 35 minutes in a 375° oven or until bread tests done when tried with a cake tester. Slide loaves out on rack to cool. Wrap in foil or saran to store.

Makes 3 loaves.

7-UP BISCUITS

2 cups sifted ALL-PURPOSE FLOUR

1 teaspoon SALT

4 teaspoons BAKING POWDER

½ cup SHORTENING

¾ cup 7-Up®

Melted MILK-FREE MARGARINE

Sift dry ingredients into bowl; cut in shortening until mixture resembles coarse corn meal. Add 7-UP all at once; stir briskly with fork until dry ingredients are evenly moistened. Turn onto lightly floured surface; knead quickly 10 times. Roll to ¾" thickness. Allow to rest five minutes. Cut with lightly floured 2-inch cutter. Arrange on baking sheet. Brush lightly with melted margarine.

Bake 10-12 minutes in a 450° oven or until golden brown. Makes 12.

CORN BREAD

1 cup sifted ALL-PURPOSE FLOUR

1 cup CORN MEAL

¼ cup SUGAR

2 teaspoons BAKING POWDER

½ teaspoon SALT

2 EGGS

¾ cup WATER

¼ cup soft MILK-FREE MARGARINE

Sift together dry ingredients into bowl. Add eggs, water, and shortening. Beat just until smooth. Pour into greased 8-inch square pan. Bake 20-25 minutes in a 425° oven.

NOTE: To make handy cakes for your toaster, cut
       bread into squares and split. Freeze.
       No need to thaw before toasting.

BANANA NUT BREAD

2 cups sifted FLOUR

1½ teaspoons BAKING POWDER

½ teaspoon BAKING SODA

2-3 BANANAS (1 cup mashed)

2 EGGS

½ cup SHORTENING

1 cup SUGAR

1½ tablespoons NON-DAIRY CREAMER

1 teaspoon LEMON JUICE

¼ teaspoon SALT

½ cup chopped NUTS

½ cup RAISINS (optional)

MIXER METHOD: Cream together shortening and sugar; add eggs and beat well. Sift together dry ingredients; add to creamed mixture alternately with the combined mashed banana, creamer, and lemon juice. Stir in nuts and raisins. Pour into well-greased 9x5x3-inch or two 8x4x3-inch loaf pans.

BLENDER METHOD: Sift dry ingredients into bowl. Blend bananas to puree; add eggs, shortening, sugar, creamer, lemon juice, and salt; blend until smooth. Pour over dry ingredients; stir just until combined. Stir in nuts and raisins. Pour into well-greased pans.

Bake 9x5x3-inch pan 45 minutes or until done in a 350° oven. Bake 8x4x3-inch pans 40 minutes or until done. Remove from pan; cool on rack.

FROSTED COFFEE COOKIES

$\frac{1}{2}$ cup SHORTENING

$\frac{1}{2}$ cup BROWN SUGAR

$\frac{1}{2}$ cup GRANULATED SUGAR

2 EGGS, well beaten

$1\frac{1}{2}$ cups FLOUR, sifted

$\frac{1}{4}$ teaspoon SALT

$\frac{1}{2}$ teaspoon BAKING SODA

$\frac{1}{2}$ teaspoon BAKING POWDER

$\frac{1}{2}$ teaspoon CINNAMON

$\frac{1}{2}$ teaspoon NUTMEG

$\frac{1}{2}$ cup cold COFFEE

$\frac{1}{2}$ teaspoon VANILLA

$\frac{1}{2}$ cup finely chopped NUTS

$\frac{1}{2}$ cup milk-free margarine

4 cups CONFECTIONERS' SUGAR

$\frac{1}{4}$ cup COFFEE

Cream shortening and sugars until light. Add eggs
and beat well. Sift together next six ingredients.
Add to first mixture alternately with the $\frac{1}{2}$ cup
coffee. Add flavoring and nuts. Spread $\frac{1}{4}$-inch
thick in two well greased $10\frac{1}{2}$x$15\frac{1}{2}$-inch shallow pans.
Bake 25 minutes in a 350° oven. Combine remaining
ingredients, creaming until smooth. Frost cookies
while hot and cut into bars when cool.

"THE BEST TREATMENT OF ALLERGY TO FOOD IS TO
AVOID THE OFFENDING FOODS IN ALL THEIR FORMS."
                        Dr. Frederic Speer
                        Speer Allergy Clinic
                        Shawnee Mission, Kan.

WALNUT BROWNIES

½ cup MILK-FREE MARGARINE

⅓ cup unsweetened COCOA or CAROB POWDER

1 teaspoon VANILLA

2 EGGS

1 cup SUGAR

¾ cup FLOUR

½ teaspoon BAKING POWDER

¼ teaspoon SALT

½ cup chopped NUTS

Melt margarine; add cocoa or carob powder and vanilla. Cool. Beat together eggs and sugar until thick and lemon-colored. Sift together dry ingredients and stir into cooled cocoa mixture. Stir in nuts. Pour into greased 8-inch square pan.

Bake 25-30 minutes in a 350° oven. Cool in pan; cut into bars.

BLUEBERRY BARS

½ cup soft MILK-FREE MARGARINE

¼ cup GRANULATED SUGAR

1 cup sifted FLOUR

½ cup sifted FLOUR

½ teaspoon BAKING POWDER

¼ teaspoon SALT

1 cup BROWN SUGAR, packed

2 EGGS, well beaten

½ teaspoon VANILLA or ALMOND

½ cup chopped NUTS

1 cup fresh BLUEBERRIES

56

Mix together first three ingredients until mixture is crumbly. Pat into bottom of greased 9x9-inch square pan. Bake 25 minutes in a 350° oven. Cool.

Meanwhile, sift together next three ingredients. Set aside. With electric mixer, gradually beat brown sugar into eggs; mix in flour mixture just until combined. Stir in flavoring and walnuts. Fold in blueberries gently. Spread evenly over cooled crust. Bake 30 minutes in a 350° oven or until browned and firm to the touch. Cool on rack. Cut into bars. Roll in CONFECTIONERS' SUGAR, if desired. Makes 2 dozen.

BUTTERSCOTCH OATMEAL COOKIES

$1\frac{1}{2}$ cups sifted FLOUR

1 teaspoon BAKING SODA

1 teaspoon SALT

1 cup BROWN SUGAR

$\frac{1}{2}$ cup GRANULATED SUGAR

1 cup MILK-FREE MARGARINE

2 EGGS

1 teaspoon VANILLA

3 cups OATMEAL

Sift together flour, baking soda, and salt. Add remaining ingredients except oatmeal; beat for two minutes. Blend in oatmeal. Shape into roll or bar (an empty plastic wrap carton makes a good "mold"). Chill overnight. Slice $\frac{1}{4}$" thick.

Bake 10-12 minutes in a 375° oven. Makes about $3\frac{1}{2}$ dozen.

COCONUT KISSES

4 EGG WHITES

½ teaspoon SALT

1¼ cups fine granulated SUGAR

1 teaspoon VANILLA

2 cups SHREDDED COCONUT

24 CANDIED CHERRIES, halved

Beat egg whites and salt until stiff. Gradually add sugar, beating well. Fold in vanilla and coconut. Drop by teaspoonfuls onto ungreased brown paper on cookie sheets. Top with cherries.

Bake 20 minutes in a 350° oven. Slip paper onto wet table. Let stand one minute. Loosen with spatula; remove to racks. Makes four dozen.

FRUIT COCKTAIL CAKE

1¼ cups FLOUR

1 cup SUGAR

1 teaspoon BAKING SODA

1 16-ounce can FRUIT COCKTAIL, undrained

1 EGG, slightly beaten

1 cup BROWN SUGAR

1 cup NUTS, chopped

1 teaspoon CINNAMON

Combine flour, sugar, and baking soda. Add fruit cocktail and egg; mix well. Pour into greased 9x13-inch pan. Combine brown sugar, nuts, and cinnamon; sprinkle over top.

Bake 45 minutes in a 325° oven. Serve warm or cold with milk-free whipped topping.

NOTE: For 6x10-inch pan, halve all ingredients except egg. Bake 35 minutes.

MAPLE CAKE

2½ cups sifted FLOUR

2 teaspoons BAKING POWDER

¾ teaspoon BAKING SODA

½ teaspoon SALT

¼ teaspoon GINGER

½ cup MILK-FREE MARGARINE

¼ cup SUGAR

2 EGGS

1 cup MAPLE SYRUP

½ cup HOT WATER

Sift together dry ingredients. Cream together margarine and sugar until light; beat in eggs and syrup until well blended. Add dry ingredients alternately with hot water blending in at low mixer speed. Pour into 2 greased, lined 8-inch round pans. Bake 30-35 minutes in a 350° oven. Cool completely on racks before removing from pans. Frost.

NOTE: To bake as CUPCAKES, fill paper baking cups in muffin pans half full. Makes 18. Bake 20 minutes.

MAPLE FROSTING

6 tablespoons MILK-FREE MARGARINE

1 teaspoon VANILLA

3 cups CONFECTIONERS' SUGAR

Dash SALT

½ cup MAPLE SYRUP

Combine all ingredients in mixer bowl and beat until mixture is of good spreading consistency. If necessary, thin with non-dairy creamer or coffee.

MOIST ORANGE CAKE

1 cup MILK-FREE MARGARINE

1 ORANGE

5 EGGS, separated

1 cup SUGAR

1 cup FLOUR

$3\frac{1}{2}$ teaspoons BAKING POWDER

2 cups WATER

1 cup SUGAR

1 tablespoon ORANGE CURACAO

Melt margarine and set aside to cool. Grate rind
from orange and extract juice (exact amount is not
important). Combine egg yolks and the 1 cup sugar
and beat well. Stir in melted margarine, rind,
juice, flour, and baking powder. Beat egg whites
until stiff and carefully fold into batter. Pour
into greased 8x10-inch or 9x9-inch pan.

Bake 10 minutes in a 375° oven; reduce temperature
to 350° and bake 30 minutes longer. Cool 15 minutes.
Meanwhile, combine the water and remaining sugar;
boil 10 minutes. Add flavoring; pour hot syrup
over cooled cake. (Flavor is best the second day.)

BANANA SPICE CUPCAKES

$\frac{1}{4}$ cup soft MILK-FREE MARGARINE

2/3 cup SUGAR

1 EGG

1 cup FLOUR

1 teaspoon BAKING POWDER

$\frac{1}{2}$ teaspoon SALT

$\frac{1}{2}$ teaspoon BAKING SODA

$\frac{1}{4}$ teaspoon CINNAMON

$\frac{1}{4}$ teaspoon NUTMEG

$\frac{1}{4}$ teaspoon ALLSPICE

$\frac{1}{2}$ cup mashed ripe BANANA

1 tablespoon non-dairy CREAMER

1 tablespoon WATER

Cream together margarine and sugar; add egg and beat until well blended. Sift together dry ingredients and spices. Combine banana, creamer, and water. Add dry ingredients to creamed mixture alternately with banana mixture and mix well. Fill paper baking cups in muffin pans half full.

Bake 20-25 minutes in a 375° oven. Makes 12.

CHOCOLATE MAYONNAISE CAKE

2 cups unsifted all-purpose FLOUR

1 cup sugar

$\frac{1}{2}$ cup unsweetened COCOA or CAROB POWDER

$1\frac{1}{2}$ teaspoons BAKING POWDER

1 teaspoon BAKING SODA

1 cup WHOLE-EGG MAYONNAISE

1 cup COLD WATER

1 teaspoon VANILLA

Sift together dry ingredients. Stir in mayonnaise. Gradually stir in water and vanilla until smooth. Pour into two greased and lined 8-inch layer pans.

Bake 30 minutes in a 350° oven or until cake tests done. Cool completely before removing from pans.

NOTE: May also be baked in one 8x12x2-inch or one 9x9x2-inch pan. No need to line pan; just cool and frost in pan. Bake 35 minutes.

COFFEE RICH POUND CAKE (R)

1½ cups SUGAR

¾ cup hydrogenated SHORTENING

6 EGGS

3¼ cups sifted CAKE FLOUR

1 tablespoon double action BAKING POWDER

1 teaspoon SALT

¾ cup COFFEE RICH®

1 teaspoon VANILLA

½ teaspoon BUTTER FLAVORING

Cream together sugar and shortening until light and fluffy. Beat in eggs, one at a time. Sift together cake flour. baking powder, and salt.

Combine Coffee Rich®, vanilla, and butter flavoring and add alternately with dry ingredients, beginning and ending with flour mixture. Pour into 3 9-inch wax paper lined or greased and floured cake pans.

Bake in 350° oven 25 minutes or until cake pulls away from sides of pan. Remove from pan. Cool. Frost as desired.

LEMON CHIFFON TARTS

1 small package LEMON PIE FILLING MIX

2 EGGS, separated

¼ cup SUGAR

6 baked TART SHELLS

Prepare pie filling mix as directed on package using the recommended amounts of sugar and water and the two egg yolks. Cool 10 minutes, stirring occasionally. Beat the two egg whites until stiff with the ¼ cup sugar. Fold into filling mix. Pour into tart shells.

BLUEBERRY TARTS

1½ tablespoons CORNSTARCH

½ cup SUGAR

½ cup WATER

3 cups BLUEBERRIES

1 tablespoon milk-free MARGARINE

6 baked TART SHELLS

Combine cornstarch, sugar, and water. Add washed blueberries and margarine. Cook and stir over medium heat until mixture is thickened and clear. Cool slightly. Fill tart shells with mixture. To serve, top with milk-free whipped topping.

COCONUT ORANGE CUSTARD PIE

3 EGGS

¾ cup SUGAR

½ cup WATER

½ cup ORANGE JUICE (preferably fresh)

2 tablespoons FLOUR

Dash SALT

½ cup SHREDDED COCONUT

1 teaspoon grated ORANGE RIND

1 8-inch UNBAKED PIE SHELL

Beat eggs well; gradually add sugar. Beat in the remaining ingredients except coconut. Pour mixture into pie shell; sprinkle coconut on top.
Bake 20 minutes in a 425° oven. Reduce temperature to 350° and bake 10 minutes longer or until knife inserted halfway between center and edge comes out clean.

NOTE: Coat pie shell with some of the egg white to prevent sogginess.

STRAWBERRY ANGEL PIE

3 EGG WHITES

1 teaspoon VANILLA

$\frac{1}{4}$ teaspoon CREAM OF TARTAR

Dash SALT

1 cup SUGAR

1 10-ounce package frozen STRAWBERRIES

1 3-ounce package STRAWBERRY GELATIN

$1\frac{1}{4}$ cups BOILING WATER

1 $4\frac{1}{2}$-ounce container COOL WHIP®

Combine egg whites, vanilla, cream of tartar, and salt; beat until frothy. Gradually add sugar, beating until very stiff peaks form and sugar is dissolved. Spoon into lightly greased 9-inch pie plate and shape into shell, swirling sides high. Bake 1 hour in a 275° oven. Turn off heat and let dry in oven with the door closed for at least two hours (or overnight).

Meanwhile, thaw strawberries; drain. Dissolve gelatin in boiling water; chill until mixture is the consistency of unbeaten egg white. Fold in thawed strawberries and Cool Whip®. Chill until mixture mounds slightly when spooned. Pile into meringue shell. Chill until firm.

HAPPY ENDINGS

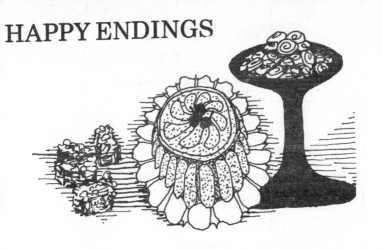

RUM MOUSSE

1 package milk-free LADY FINGERS

3 EGGS, separated

$\frac{1}{2}$ cup SUGAR

1 9-ounce container COOL WHIP®

1 teaspoon VANILLA

2 tablespoons light RUM

Wash and dry eggs well before separating; bring to room temperature. Arrange lady fingers in bottom of 8x8x2 pan. Beat egg yolks adding sugar slowly and beating until thick and lemon colored. Beat egg whites until stiff. Fold yolks into whites, then fold in Cool Whip®. Add flavorings and pour mixture over lady fingers. Sprinkle with shaved unsweetened chocolate, if desired.

Freeze 4 hours or more but remove from freezer a few minutes before serving.

CHEESELESS CHEESECAKE

1¼ cups GRAHAM CRACKER CRUMBS

¼ cup MILK-FREE MARGARINE, melted

1 tablespoon SUGAR

½ teaspoon CINNAMON

½ cup boiling WATER

1 1-oz. package LEMON GELATIN

2 tablespoons LEMON JUICE

½ teaspoon grated LEMON RIND

2 cups crumbled TOFU*

1 10-oz. container DESSERT WHIP, thawed

Press excess moisture from tofu; crumble and measure. Place on paper towel and let any additional moisture drain while preparing remaining ingredients. Combine crumbs, margarine, sugar, and cinnamon and press onto bottom of 8" round spring form pan or cake pan. Set aside. Pour boiling water into blender container, add gelatin and blend until dissolved. Add lemon juice, rind, and part of the tofu. Blend until smooth. Add remaining tofu gradually; continue to blend until smooth. Pour into large bowl. Add dessert whip and combine with spatula or mixer at low speed. Pour over crust. Chill until set. For a special treat, serve with sweetened fresh or frozen strawberries.

NOTE: If you prefer not to use frozen dessert whip, you may add ¼ cup non-dairy liquid creamer to the blended ingredients and substitute a meringue made of four egg whites, stiffly beaten with ½ cup sugar and ½ teaspoon vanilla, for the dessert whip. This will make a lighter, less rich cheesecake.

ORANGE-PINEAPPLE TAPIOCA

½ cup SUGAR

3 tablespoons TAPIOCA

¼ teaspoon SALT

1¾ cups ORANGE JUICE (about)

2 tablespoons MILK-FREE MARGARINE

1 EGG YOLK

1 EGG WHITE

2 tablespoons SUGAR

1 8-oz. can CRUSHED PINEAPPLE

½ teaspoon grated LEMON RIND

Drain pineapple, reserving liquid. Add enough orange juice to make 2 cups. Combine sugar, tapioca, salt, and egg yolk in pan. Add juices and margarine; let stand 5 minutes. Cook and stir over medium heat until mixture comes to a boil; stir in lemon rind. Beat egg white with the 2 tablespoons of sugar until peaks form. Gradually add hot mixture to beaten white, stirring quickly just until blended. Fold in pineapple. Cool 20 minutes. Stir. Chill.

GRANOLA APPLE CRISP

1 cup GRANOLA*

½ cup FLOUR

1 cup SUGAR

1 teaspoon CINNAMON

½ cup MILK-FREE MARGARINE

4 cups sliced APPLES, pared

Rub together flour, sugar, cinnamon, and margarine; mix in Granola. Place apples in greased 8x8x2-inch baking dish. Drop Granola mixture over apples by spoonfuls. Bake 40 minutes in a 350° oven.

ORANGE VELVET SHERBET (R)

1 quart COFFEE RICH®

$\frac{1}{2}$ cup LEMON JUICE

$3\frac{1}{2}$ cups ORANGE JUICE (1- 6 oz. can
   frozen orange juice reconstituted)

3 cups SUGAR

1 tablespoon unflavored GELATIN

$\frac{1}{4}$ cup COLD WATER

Blend together Coffee Rich®, citrus juices, and
sugar until sugar is dissolved. Dissolve gelatin
in cold water; melt over hot water bath. Beating,
add to Coffee Rich® mixture until well blended.

Freeze until firm using 8 parts ice to 1 part salt.

PHILADELPHIA ICE CREAM (R)

1 quart COFFEE RICH®

$\frac{3}{4}$ cup SUGAR

1 teaspoon VANILLA

1 pinch SALT

Mix all ingredients to dissolve sugar. Freeze
until firm using 8 parts ice to 1 part salt.

NOTE: For COFFEE ICE CREAM, dissolve $1\frac{1}{2}$ table-
        spoons instant coffee in 2 tablespoons
        hot water and add to ice cream mixture.
        For MAPLE NUT ICE CREAM, add 1 cup finely
        chopped nuts and substitute maple flavor-
        ing for vanilla in ice cream mix.
        For PEPPERMINT STICK ICE CREAM, substitute
        $\frac{1}{2}$ pound crushed peppermint stick candy for
        sugar and vanilla.

NOTE: These recipes freeze equally well in the in-
        freezer electric ice cream maker using only
        24 ounces of the mixture for each batch.

BUTTERSCOTCH SWIRL ICE CREAM

$\frac{1}{4}$ cup BROWN SUGAR

2 tablespoons milk-free MARGARINE

2 tablespoons DARK CORN SYRUP

3 tablespoons non-dairy CREAMER

Combine all ingredients; boil 2 minutes. Cool.
Fold into 1 pint VANILLA PHILADELPHIA ICE CREAM*
for marbled effect. Freeze.

EASY BAVARIAN (GF)

1 3-oz. package JELL-O®, any red flavor

$\frac{1}{4}$ cup SUGAR

1 cup BOILING WATER

$1\frac{1}{2}$ cups thawed COOL WHIP®

Dissolve Jell-o® and sugar in boiling water. Add
1 cup cold water. Chill until slightly thickened.
Blend Cool Whip® into gelatin. Chill in 1-quart
or 6-8 individual molds until firm. Unmold and
garnish with additional Cool Whip®.
Makes 6-8 servings.

JEWELLED BAVARIAN CREAM

1 3-oz. package JELL-O®, any red flavor

1 cup BOILING WATER

$\frac{1}{2}$ cup non-dairy CREAMER

Dissolve gelatin in boiling water. Combine $\frac{1}{2}$ cup
of the gelatin mixture with the $\frac{1}{2}$ cup non-dairy
creamer. Chill in small mixing bowl. Add cold
water to remaining gelatin to make $1\frac{1}{4}$ cups. Pour
into 8" square pan and chill until very firm.
Beat creamy portion with mixer until fluffy. Dice
clear portion into small cubes and fold into the
cream. Spoon into serving dishes and chill.
Makes 4 servings.

8-MINUTE CHOCOLATE FUDGE

2 cups granulated SUGAR

2 squares UNSWEETENED CHOCOLATE

Dash SALT

$\frac{1}{4}$ cup WATER

$\frac{1}{4}$ cup non-dairy CREAMER

2 tablespoons milk-free MARGARINE

1 teaspoon VANILLA

$\frac{1}{2}$ cup WALNUTS, chopped (optional)

Combine sugar, chocolate, salt, water and creamer in saucepan and place over HIGH heat. Bring to boil; lower to MEDIUM heat. Boil stirring occasionally until ingredients are blended. This should take four minutes at the most; color will look more even. Remove from heat; immediately add margarine and vanilla. Beat with mixer until batter starts to thicken; quickly add nuts and pour into shallow, greased 5x9-inch pan. Cool.

EASY PENUCHE

1 pound BROWN SUGAR (2$\frac{1}{3}$ cups)

$\frac{1}{2}$ cup non-dairy CREAMER

$\frac{1}{4}$ cup WATER

2 tablespoons MILK-FREE MARGARINE

1 teaspoon VANILLA

$\frac{1}{2}$ cup WALNUTS, chopped

Combine brown sugar, creamer, and water; stir well to break up any lumps of sugar. Cook as directed above except allow to cool five minutes before beating and use shallow 8x8-inch pan. Mark in squares before completely cool.

NOTE: Once you get the "feel" of these recipes, you'll be able to satisfy sweet tooth cravings with fudge that rivals the candy thermometer, kneaded kind quickly and easily.

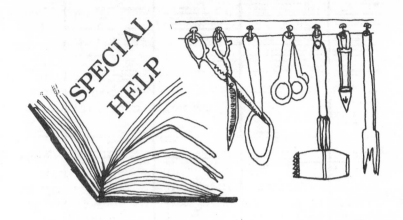

SPECIAL HELP

... for milk-free diets

COCONUT MILK: Fresh coconut milk or canned coconut juice, usually available in 8-ounce cans.
(If allergic, avoid brands containing sodium
caseinate.) Use for baking or in beverages.

"NON-DAIRY" LIQUID CREAMERS: (If allergic, avoid
brands containing sodium caseinate.) May be
used successfully in almost any recipe except
custards, puddings, and delicate cakes. Use
full strength for coffee and rich cream sauce.
Dilute two parts creamer to one part water for
regular cream sauce, hot cereals, or making
cream pies and dessert sauces. Keep some on
hand, already diluted with an equal part
water, for general use as you would milk -
in tapioca, scrambled eggs, milk shakes, or
poured over cold cereals. Diluted this way,
"non-dairy" liquid creamer has the same number
of calories as whole milk but not the nutritional value.

SOY MILK SUBSTITUTES: Isomil, Neo-Mullsoy, Pro-
 Sobee, Soyalac, Similac. Instant powdered
 soybean which can be mixed like dried milk is
 available in most health food stores. All
 have a stronger flavor than milk but can be
 used for drinking or in cooking and baking
 and have a nutritional value comparable to
 milk.

ADJUSTING RECIPES: While the fat and sugar content of the "non-dairy" creamers make them
 unsatisfactory for delicate cakes, you may be
 able to continue using some of your favorite
 cake recipes by substituting a combination of
 water, extra egg, and oil for the milk called
 for in the recipe. Break one egg in measuring
 cup; add two tablespoons oil; fill cup with
 water to make two cups. Blend ingredients
 well and measure out amount needed to replace
 milk in recipe.

CHOCOLATE SUBSTITUTE: Carob powder, processed
 from the nutritious Carob bean, is available
 as a flavorful substitute for cocoa in baking
 or beverages. It can be found at most health
 food stores but be sure to buy the plain
 "powder" rather than the drink "mix" which
 contains dried milk. Use in the same propor-
 tions as you would cocoa. As a substitute
 for unsweetened chocolate, use 3 tablespoons
 carob powder and 1 tablespoon milk-free margarine for each 1-ounce square.

"WE MUST CAUTION PERSONS WITH MILK ALLERGIES
THAT SINCE ALLERGIES ARE SO HIGHLY INDIVIDUA-
LIZED AND CAN BE AREAS OF EXTREME SENSITIVITY,
WE RECOMMEND THAT THEY EVALUATE THESE PRODUCTS
WITH THEIR ALLERGIST BEFORE MAKING ANY FINAL
DECISION ON USING THEM."
                              Rich Products Corporation

TOFU: THE VERSATILE SOY CHEESE

If you've wondered how to satisfy the need for calcium in your diet, you may find the answer in tofu, the "cheese" made from curds of soybean milk.

Unlike soy milk, which has a stronger flavor than we have been accustomed to in cow's milk, tofu is almost tasteless. For this reason, it needs careful preparation and seasoning but it can be substituted for cheese, used to extend meat or fish dishes, and used in salads, sandwich fillings or desserts. Its' nutritional value makes it a boon for anyone on a milk-free diet.

Tofu can be purchased fresh in some vegetable markets (where you'll probably find the creamy looking cakes floating in a tub of water) or in health food stores. It is also available canned or vacuum sealed in plastic containers. The method of packaging will determine how long it will stay fresh in your refrigerator or pantry but, once opened, will normally remain fresh for about a week. To ensure that it retains its mild flavor, it should be stored in a container of water in the refrigerator and the water changed daily.

The molded cakes of fresh tofu usually weigh between 6 and 8 ounces while most canned or vacuum sealed packages come in a one pound size. Japanese style tofu is less compact, often lighter in color (like cottage cheese) than the Chinese style which is pressed into firmer, drier cakes.

When preparing to use tofu, it is best to press it gently first to remove as much moisture from it as you can. Just slice, cube, or crumble it as the recipe directs and weight it down. In 15 or 20 minutes the excess moisture will be absorbed by the towels and it will be ready for use.

While there are only a few tofu recipes in this cookbook, its' uses are almost endless. The traditional Japanese way is to dice it and serve it with a variety of highly seasoned sauces for dipping. In our own kitchen, we like to marinate the cubes briefly in a spicy salad dressing, chill well, and serve in tossed salad. And, of course, you'll find dozens of ideas - starting with Sukiyaki - in any good Oriental cookbook.

Brands vary in texture and flavor so, if you aren't "turned on" by your first venture with tofu, try again - the nutrients make it worthwhile. To emphasize its' value, we've included the following comparison chart:

NUTRIENT	3.5% fat WHOLE MILK 2 cups	Uncreamed COTTAGE CHEESE 1 pound	Soybean TOFU 1 pound
. . . .Percentage*of U.S. RDA. . . .			
VITAMIN A:	12	1	-
VITAMIN B1:	8	9	17
VITAMIN B2:	50	75	8
CALCIUM:	30	41	58
IRON:	-	10	48
CALORIES:	(320)	(390)	(327)

*Rounded to nearest %

-Negligible or less than 1%

MAKING MILK EASIER TO DIGEST

There are products on the market now that may make it possible for you to drink milk IF your problem is simple lactose intolerance. However, if you are allergic to milk or suffer from galactosemia, these treated milk products can't help you. If you are diabetic, or have had milk removed from your diet for other medical reasons, you should consult your doctor first.

Lact-Aid® is a lactase enzyme preparation which makes milk digestible for persons who are unable to digest lactose, the complex natural milk sugar. Lact-Aid® does for you what your own body can't do if you are lactose-intolerant; that is, separate the lactose into the more digestible sugars, glucose and galactose.

Lact-Aid® is a powder which, when added to milk, can hydrolyze a predictable level of lactose before the milk is consumed. The longer the blended milk stands in the refrigerator, the higher the level of lactose conversion. After twenty-four hours of blending, the milk has had about 70% of the original lactose converted to the more easily digested galactose and glucose. The conversion level can reach 90% after three or four days in the refrigerator. Higher levels of conversion can also be achieved by adding more Lact-Aid® or by heating the milk according to the instructions provided.

Lact-Aid® treated milk will taste a little sweeter than untreated milk and will also be more perishable. It should always be handled carefully and refrigerated promptly. The treated milk can be used for cooking and baking. Lact-Aid® treated milk may also be cultured but Lact-Aid® cannot be used to treat other dairy products, such as cheese, yogurt, or buttermilk. Since it is an enzyme that can be destroyed by too much heat, you should follow instructions for its use carefully.

Lact-Aid® is produced by the SugarLo Company. Anyone wishing more information can write the company at the address shown in the "Where to Write ..." section on page 89. They'll be pleased to send you two trial packets for 25¢ in coin or stamps.

If your digestive problems have you walking by the supermarket dairy department without stopping, you may not know that some stores now carry milk that is fortified with the bacteria, "Lactobacillus Acidophilus". This product is sold under the trademark "Sweet Acidophilus".

While apparently there are no wholly conclusive research findings at this point, preliminary indications are that this product may ease some of the common problems induced by lactose intolerance; intestinal cramps and diarrhea, for example.

The introduction of Lactobacillus Acidophilus to the human body is not new. The same bacteria is used in yogurt cultures and all fermented milk products, such as buttermilk.

Like all dietary changes, check this one with your doctor first since it is likely that it can only be of help to those who are only mildly lactose-intolerant.

A WORD ABOUT NUTRITION

When you start your milk-free diet, you'll want to ask your doctor's advice about possible nutritional deficiencies that may result from giving up dairy products. He may prescribe supplements or he may recommend seeing that the rest of your diet is well balanced. Following is a list of the vitamins and minerals that are most likely to be deficient in a milk-free diet and the alternative food sources from which these nutrients may be obtained.

You'll notice that the figure in the last column on page 78 shows the percentage of the U.S. Recommended Daily Allowance provided by a specific size portion of that food. Actually, not all people need 100% of the U.S. RDA for each nutrient every day. The U.S. Recommended Daily Allowances are the amounts used as standards in nutrition labeling; your personal needs are determined by your age, sex, and overall physical condition.

A young child, for example, may need only 80% of the U.S. RDA for calcium while a teenager or nursing woman would require 120%. The need for iron varies greatly, too, with women needing 100% until after menopause whereas 60% of the U.S. RDA will suffice for most adult males.

This information is presented primarily to enable you to compensate for milk-free diet related deficiencies. Follow your doctor's recommendations as to your individual requirements and use the list to fulfill those needs with wholesome foods. Nutritionists have found that the interaction among nutrients is such that the lack of any one can diminish the ability of the body to utilize the others. So, try to keep your diet as well balanced as possible.

77

NUTRIENT	FOOD SOURCE	PROVIDES (% of RDA)
VITAMIN A:	*Liver,beef,3oz.	910
	Carrots,1c.diced,cooked	330
	Spinach,1c.cooked	290
	Sweet potato,1 med.	180
	Cantaloupe,½ of 5" melon	180
	Apricots,dried,cooked,1c.	150
	Prune juice,1c.	30
	Asparagus,1c.cooked	25
VITAMIN B1: (Thiamin)	Pork chop,lean,3oz.	60
	Sunflower seeds,¼c.	47
	*Peas,1c.cooked	30
	*Beans,Lima,1c.cooked	20
	Asparagus,1c.cooked	15
	Rice,1c.cooked	14
	Avocado,1c.cubed	10
VITAMIN B2: (Riboflavin)	*Liver,beef,3oz.	210
	Avocado,1c.cubed	20
	Mushrooms,1c.raw	20
	Broccoli,1c.cooked	17
	Brussels sprouts,1c.	15
	Asparagus,1c.cooked	15
CALCIUM:	Sardines,drained,3oz.	35
	Almonds,shelled,1c.	35
	Tofu,bean curd,½lb.	29
	Turnip greens,1c.cooked	25
	Rhubarb,1c.cooked	20
	Salmon,3oz.	20
	Spinach,1c.cooked	15
	Broccoli,1c.cooked	15
	*Beans,Lima,1c.cooked	8
IRON:	Prune juice,1c.	60
	*Liver,beef,3oz.	40
	Tofu,bean curd,½lb.	24
	Spinach,1c.cooked	20
	Sunflower seeds,¼c.	15

*If able to tolerate.

Granola cereals are a popular favorite but most
commercial brands contain some non-fat dry milk.
Here's . . .

HOMEMADE GRANOLA

4 cups OATMEAL (not instant)

$\frac{1}{2}$ cup WHEAT GERM

1 cup SUNFLOWER SEEDS

$\frac{3}{4}$ cup NUTS, chopped

$\frac{3}{4}$ cup DATES and/or RAISINS

$\frac{1}{2}$ cup CORN OIL

$\frac{1}{2}$ cup HONEY or BROWN SUGAR

2 teaspoons VANILLA

Combine oatmeal and wheat germ in large bowl.
Mix together oil, honey or brown sugar, and
vanilla. Drizzle over cereals and mix well;
spread on greased baking sheet. Bake 45 minutes in a 225° oven. Stir in remaining ingredients; bake 15 minutes longer.

NOTE: To vary GRANOLA to suit your own tastes,
change ingredients or amounts. Other
nuts or dried fruits can be used, bran
rolled whole wheat, sesame seeds, coconut, or almost any grain, seed, nut, or
dried fruit you have on hand.

. . . Being sensitive to milk doesn't mean you have to miss all of those casseroles made with commercial condensed Cream of Mushroom Soup. Here's the answer . . .

CREAM-OF-MUSHROOM SOUP SUBSTITUTE

$\frac{1}{4}$ cup minced ONION

2 tablespoons minced CELERY

1 clove GARLIC, minced

3 tablespoons MILK-FREE MARGARINE

$\frac{1}{2}$ pound fresh MUSHROOMS, chopped

$\frac{1}{4}$ cup FLOUR

1 cup CHICKEN or BEEF BROTH
(or 1 cube dissolved in hot water)

$1\frac{1}{2}$ cups non-dairy CREAMER

$\frac{1}{2}$ teaspoon BASIL

$\frac{3}{4}$ teaspoon SALT

Saute onion, celery, and garlic in margarine until soft. Add mushrooms and brown lightly. Sprinkle flour over, stirring constantly and cooking until all flour is blended in. Gradually add broth, seasonings, and creamer. Bring to boil slowly and simmer two minutes, stirring constantly.

Makes about $2\frac{1}{2}$ cups or the equivalent of two cans of commercial Cream of Mushroom Soup.

NOTE: Recipe doubles easily if you want to make extra for the freezer. Try freezing $1\frac{1}{4}$ cup single recipe portions in plastic sandwich boxes. When solid, pop out of box, wrap in foil and label. Boxes are ready for re-use. To thaw: Place in saucepan with liquid required for recipe. Heat slowly over low flame or in double boiler.

SEASONED BREAD CRUMBS

Stale MILK-FREE ITALIAN BREAD

1 teaspoon MARJORAM or OREGANO

½ teaspoon THYME

½ teaspoon PAPRIKA

Grate bread in blender or on hand grater. Add remaining ingredients to 1½ cups of the bread crumbs combining thoroughly by shaking well or whirling in blender. Save any leftover crumbs for PLAIN BREAD CRUMBS.

MINI-CROUTONS

4 cups ¼" cubes fresh MILK-FREE BREAD
                (about 5 slices white
                    and 3 slices rye)

2 tablespoons OIL

1 tablespoon DRIED PARSLEY

¾ teaspoon GARLIC SALT

1 teaspoon DRIED MINCED ONION

½ teaspoon EACH: OREGANO and PAPRIKA,

¼ teaspoon EACH: THYME, BASIL, PEPPER

Toast bread cubes in shallow baking pan or on cookie sheet 30 minutes in a 300° oven. Cool slightly. Drizzle with oil; stir in spices, mixing well. Cool before storing in airtight containers. Sprinkle on salads.

FRESH CROUTONS

2 cups ½-inch WHITE MILK-FREE BREAD cubes

2 tablespoons OIL

1 clove GARLIC (optional)

Use firm type bread if available. Heat oil in heavy skillet; saute bread cubes with garlic over medium heat until golden on all sides. Remove garlic. Drain cubes on paper towels.

. . . Here's a delicious way to sneak a few extra nutrients into a variety of pastry recipes. No one will suspect your "secret ingredient". . .

"CHEESE" PASTRY

1 cup MILK-FREE MARGARINE

1 cup TOFU, crumbled

2 cups sifted FLOUR

1 tablespoon SUGAR

$\frac{1}{4}$ teaspoon SALT

Drain tofu well to remove excess moisture. Cream the margarine and tofu together until smooth and creamy. Sift together remaining ingredients; work into creamed mixture with pastry cutter or wooden spoon. Mold into a ball; wrap in plastic wrap and chill several hours.

COOKIES: Roll about 1/8" thick; cut into 2$\frac{1}{2}$" squares. Place a teaspoonful of tart jam or preserves (cherry or raspberry is particularly good) in the center of each square. Fold corners to center to enclose filling. Bake 15 minutes in a 425° oven or until lightly browned. Cool. Sprinkle with confectioners' sugar. Almost like mini "pop-tarts" and nutritious enough to serve for breakfast.

MINI-MEAT PIES: Brown $\frac{1}{2}$ pound lean ground beef with 1 small chopped onion. Add $\frac{1}{2}$ teaspoon salt, $\frac{1}{4}$ teaspoon marjoram, a dash of salt and 1 teaspoon dried parsley. (If filling is very moist, add 1 tablespoon bread crumbs or flour.) Cut rolled dough into 4" squares; place about 1 tablespoon filling on each. Fold in half diagonally and press edges with fork tines to seal. Bake as for Cookies.

WHITE SAUCE

1 tablespoon MILK-FREE MARGARINE

¼ cup FLOUR

¼ teaspoon SALT

Dash PEPPER

½ cup WATER

1 cup liquid non-dairy CREAMER

Melt butter in saucepan; blend in flour, salt, pepper, and water. Add creamer. Cook and stir until thickened and sauce comes to a boil.

NOTE: The proportion of margarine to flour is reduced to compensate for the higher fat content of the non-dairy creamer.

To make a thinner sauce, reduce the flour to 2 tablespoons.

BEER BATTER FOR DEEP FRYING

1 cup SELF-RISING FLOUR

2 EGG YOLKS, beaten

2 EGG WHITES

½ cup FLAT BEER

Combine flour, egg yolks, and beer; stir until batter is smooth. Chill 3-12 hours. Beat egg whites until soft peaks form: fold into batter.

May be used to deep fry chicken, fish, seafood, or vegetables (try whole mushrooms, onion rings, sticks of zucchini or eggplant).

TOFU "SOUR CREAM"

5 tablespoons NON-DAIRY CREAMER

1 tablespoon LEMON JUICE

1 cup crumbled TOFU

Put ingredients in blender container. Blend
until smooth. May be used as a substitute for
sour cream in molded salads or well-seasoned
dips.

. . . And a variety of salad dressings for those
times when you can't find a commercial product
that doesn't contain blended spices or mono-
sodium glutamate. . .

BOILED SALAD DRESSING

1 EGG, slightly beaten

$\frac{1}{3}$ cup SUGAR

$1\frac{1}{2}$ tablespoons FLOUR

$\frac{1}{2}$ teaspoon DRY MUSTARD

2/3 cup WATER

$\frac{1}{3}$ cup VINEGAR

2 tablespoons milk-free MARGARINE

1 teaspoon SALT

$\frac{1}{4}$ teaspoon PEPPER

Combine all ingredients; boil until thickened.
Good for potato salad; for best flavor, combine
ingredients while still warm; chill. (Crisp,
fried bacon, crumbled makes a complementary
addition.) May also be beaten into mayonnaise
to vary the flavor or decrease the proportion
of oil.

BLENDER MAYONNAISE

1 EGG

1/8 teaspoon WHITE PEPPER

1/8 teaspoon PAPRIKA

$\frac{1}{4}$ teaspoon DRY MUSTARD

1 teaspoon SUGAR

1 tablespoon LEMON JUICE

1 tablespoon SALAD VINEGAR

$\frac{1}{2}$ teaspoon SALT

1 cup PURE CORN OIL

Have all ingredients at room temperature. Put egg, seasonings, lemon juice, vinegar and $\frac{1}{4}$ cup of the oil in blender container, cover and turn to blend. Immediately remove center cap and pour in remaining oil in a slow, steady stream. If necessary, stop blender occasionally and use rubber spatula to keep mixture moving into blades. Process until thick and smooth.

NOTE: Homemade mayonnaise does not keep as long as commercial mayonnaise so plan to use within a week and keep refrigerated.

TARTAR SAUCE

$\frac{1}{2}$ cup MAYONNAISE*

1 teaspoon DRIED PARSLEY

2 teaspoons SWEET PICKLE RELISH

2 teaspoons CAPERS

1 teaspoon minced ONION

Combine all ingredients; chill to blend flavors.

PLAIN SALAD DRESSING

$\frac{3}{4}$ cup SALAD OIL

$\frac{1}{4}$ cup VINEGAR or LEMON JUICE

$\frac{1}{2}$ teaspoon SALT

Dash PEPPER

1 tablespoon SUGAR

1 clove GARLIC, mashed

Combine ingredients in jar and shake well.

ITALIAN SALAD DRESSING

1 tablespoon SUGAR

1 teaspoon SALT

$\frac{1}{2}$ teaspoon DRY MUSTARD

$\frac{1}{2}$ teaspoon PAPRIKA

$\frac{1}{2}$ teaspoon OREGANO

1 clove GARLIC, minced

$\frac{1}{4}$ cup ONION, finely chopped

$\frac{1}{4}$ cup WINE VINEGAR

$\frac{1}{4}$ cup CATSUP

$\frac{3}{4}$ cup SALAD OIL

Combine dry ingredients in jar and mix well. Add remaining ingredients; shake well. Chill.

. . . And for fruit salads . . .

FRESH STRAWBERRY DRESSING

$\frac{3}{4}$ cup sliced ripe STRAWBERRIES

2 tablespoons LIGHT CORN SYRUP

$\frac{1}{2}$ cup MAYONNAISE

Mash strawberries together with corn syrup. Add mayonnaise, stirring until well blended. Chill.

BASIC COOKBOOK RECIPES TO LOOK FOR

. . . A word about the recipes in this book.
Like any specialty cookbook, this one was created
to serve a special need: creamy desserts and
saucy foods that can satisfy that desire for
something rich and "gooey" that seems to be even
more urgent when you are on a milk-free diet and
know it's a "no-no". Therefore, this is not a
complete cookbook and lacks many of the recipes
that make up the bulk of plain, nutritious,
everyday cooking. Milk-free cooking requires
more "cooking from scratch" so here are a few
suggestions for recipes found in most cookbooks;
usually they are milk-free or easily adjusted.

BAKED BEANS: substitute maple syrup for molasses.

BREADS AND ROLLS: Italian, potato water, fruit/nut
    tea loaves, breadsticks.

CAKES: Angel food, sponge, applesauce or fruit.

CANDIES: Marshmallows, nougats, fruit jellies,
    popcorn balls, divinity.

COOKIES: Most require so little milk that fruit
    juice or "non-dairy" creamer can be substituted.

FROSTINGS: "Seven Minute" or marshmallow, fruit
    glazes. Use milk-free margarine and juice,
    coffee, or "non-dairy" creamer in Buttercream
    type frostings.

FRUIT: Pies, pastries, cobblers, baked apples,
    stewed fruit, salads, frozen ices.

MEAT LOAVES: Substitute tomato juice, bouillion, or chopped, canned tomatoes for milk. Use milk-free bread, oatmeal, or tapioca.

PIES: Lemon or Orange Meringue, some Chiffon pies, most fruit pies.

SALADS: Fruit, vegetable, "Three Bean", coleslaw with mayonnaise, carrot and raisin, Waldorf. For "chef's salad", substitute quartered hard boiled eggs or milk-free bologna for the cheese. Molded gelatin salads using fruits or vegetables.

SANDWICHES: Chicken, tuna, milk-free cold cuts, barbecued meats.

STUFFINGS: Rice, Kasha, or milk-free cornbread as a change from milk-free bread.

TAPIOCA: made with fruit juice.

ZABAGLIONE: A delicious milk-free dessert. Good served over fresh fruit or berries.

THINK OF YOURSELF AS THE SHERLOCK HOLMES OF THE SUPERMARKET AND WRITE TO THE FOOD MANUFACTURER WHEN YOU'RE UNCERTAIN ABOUT AN INGREDIENT. IT WILL GIVE YOU THE INFORMATION YOU NEED AND GIVE HIM AN AWARENESS OF THE IMPORTANCE OF NOT ALLOWING ANY "HIDDEN" INGREDIENTS IN HIS PRODUCTS.

WHERE TO WRITE FOR PRODUCT INFORMATION

BEST FOODS DIV. OF CPC INTERNATIONAL, Consumer Service Dept., International Plaza, Englewood Cliffs, NJ 17632

BEATRICE FOODS CO., 120 South LaSalle St., Chicago, IL 60603

BORDEN, INC., Customer Service, 180 E. Broad St., Columbus, OH 43125 Attention: Anna Hunter (Cremora)

CAMPBELL SOUP CO., General Offices, Camden, NJ 08101

CENTRAL SOYA COMPANY, INC., 1300 Fort Wayne National Bank Bldg., Fort Wayne, IN 46802 (Censoya, Soyamix).

FEARN SOYA FOODS, 4520 James Place, Melrose Park, IL 60160 (Soya Powder and Granules, Soy/o Mixes)

GENERAL FOODS, Consumer Center, 250 North St., White Plains, NY 10625

GENERAL MILLS, Nutrition Service, P.O. Box 1113, Minneapolis, MN 55540

H.J. HEINZ CO., Home Economics Dept., P.O. Box 57 Pittsburgh, PA 15230

HUDSON PHARMACEUTICAL CORPORATION, 21 Henderson Drive, West Caldwell, NJ 07006

KEEBLER CO., 677 Larch Ave., Elmhurst, IL 60126

LAWRY'S FOODS, 568 San Fernando Rd., Los Angeles, CA 90065

LEDERLE LABS, Product Information, Middletown Rd., Pearl River, NY 10965 (Pharmaceuticals)

LIBBY, McNEIL & LIBBY, 200 S. Michigan Ave., Chicago, IL 60604

MITCHELL FOODS, Fredonia, NY 14063 (Perx and
Poly Perx)

NABISCO, INC., 195 River Rd., East Hanover, NJ
07936

PFIZER, INC. 235 E. 42nd St., New York, NY 10017
Attention: Dr. Wroblewski (Pharmaceuticals)

PILLSBURY CO., Dept. of Nutrition, Pillsbury
Bldg., Minneapolis, MN 55402

QUAKER OATS CO., Consumer Services, Chicago, IL
60654

RICH PRODUCTS CORPORATION, P.O. Box 245, 1145
Niagara St., Buffalo, NY 14240 (Coffee Rich)

STANDARD BRANDS CORP., 625 Madison Ave., New
York, NY 10022

SUGARLO COMPANY, 3540 Atlantic Ave., P.O. Box
1017, Atlantic City, NJ 08404 (Lact-Aid)

SYNTEX LABORATORIES, INC. 3401 Hillsview Ave.,
Palo Alto, CA 94304 (Mullsoy)

CHICKEN

Chicken-Macaroni Casserole	33
Skillet Herb Chicken	34
Versatile Baked Chicken	32

COOKIES

Blueberry Bars	56
Breakfast Cookies	17
Butterscotch Oatmeal Cookies	57
Coconut Kisses	58
Filled "Cheese" Cookies	82
Frosted Coffee Cookies	55
Walnut Brownies	56

DESSERTS

Butterscotch Swirl Ice Cream	69
Cheeseless Cheesecake	66
Easy Bavarian	69
Easy Penuche	70
Eight-Minute Choco-late Fudge	70
Jewelled Bavarian Cream	69
Orange-Pineapple Tapioca	67
Orange Velvet Sherbet	68
Philadelphia Ice Cream	68
Rum Mousse	65

EGGS

Herbed Mushroom Omelet	38
Puffed Omelet	18
Spanish Omelet	38

FISH, SEAFOOD

Creamy Scallop Casserole	35
Crunchy Tuna Bake	35
Oven Fried Filets	36
Seven Seas Casserole	36
Tuna-Tofu Loaf	37

MISCELLANEOUS

Beer Batter	83
Granola, Homemade	79
Tofu "Sour Cream"	84
White Sauce	83

PIES, PASTRIES

Blueberry Tarts	63
"Cheese" Pastry	82
Coconut Orange Custard Pie	63
Lemon Chiffon Tarts	62
Strawberry Angel Pie	64

PORK

Pork Skillet Dinner	34

SALAD DRESSINGS

Boiled Salad Dressing 84
Fresh Strawberry
       Dressing 86
Italian Dressing 86
Mayonnaise, Blender 85
Plain Dressing 86
Tartar Sauce 85

SALADS

Cherry Salad 49
Cranberry Mold 48
Ham-Rice Salad 48
Pineapple-Carrot
      Salad 50
Pineapple-Lime Salad 49
Sweet 'n Sour Cole-
      slaw 50
Tuna-Macaroni Salad 47

SOUPS

Clam Chowder 47
Cream of Celery Soup 46
Cream-of-Mushroom
  Soup Substitute 80
Cream of Tomato Soup 46
Speedy Hamburger Soup 45

VEGETABLES AND
SIDE DISHES

Baked Bean Casserole 39
Baked Carrots 40
Barbecue Rice 43
Green Beans Lucette 41
Noodle Ring 44
San Antonio Spinach
      Pudding 42
Savory Lemon Rice 43
Savory Oven Baked
      Rice 42
Savory Tomatoes 40
Tofu Manicotti 31
Zucchini Provencal 41

An order form follows for your convenience in ordering "LIVING ... WITHOUT MILK" for friends or relatives who may share your problem.

For more information on the food sources of nutrients, we recommend NUTRI-DIET™, a program which will enable you to plan your own diet for health maintenance or weight loss.

The NUTRI-DIET™ Guide is a "how-to" booklet, chock-full of valuable information, tables, and guidelines. NUTRI-DIARY™, the companion booklet, enables you to tally your daily intake of calories, carbohydrates, and eight basic nutrients almost automatically. Both booklets come packaged in an attractive pocket or purse-sized vinyl case, for easy and discreet reference.

Order Form

Betterway Publications
240 East 27th Street, Box 7G
New York, NY 10016
Yes, please RUSH the following items:

_____ NUTRI-DIET™/NUTRI-DIARY™(s)
with vinyl case @ $3.95 ea.   _____

_____ LIVING...WITHOUT MILK @ $3.95 ea. _____

Handling (any number of items)   70¢

Total Amount Enclosed: _____

NAME _____

ADDRESS _____

CITY _____ STATE _____ ZIP _____